Your *Guide to* Healthy Hormones

Daniel Kalish, D.C.

Your Guide to Healthy Hormones

By Daniel Kalish, D.C.

Published by:

The Natural Path
2105 Industrial Court
Vista, CA 92081

Dr. Kalish's Office:

800.616.7708
760.597.0808 fax

www.drkalish.com
www.yourguidetohealthyhormones.com

Printed in the United States of America
First Edition

ISBN: 0-9768628-0-8
Paperback $14.95

Book Designed by Cheryl Tsai

Warning – Disclaimer

The Natural Path has designed this book to provide information in regard to the subject matter covered. It is sold with the understanding that the publisher and the author are not liable for the misconception of misuse of the information provided. Every effort has been made to make this book as complete and as accurate as possible. The purpose of this book is to educate. The author and The Natural Path shall have neither liability nor responsibility to any person or entity with respect to any loss, damage, or injury caused or alleged to be caused directly or indirectly by the information contained in this book. The information presented herein is in no way intended as a substitute for medical counseling.

Dedication

This book is dedicated to the memory of my father, Richard A. Kalish. I grew up from an early age falling asleep every night to the sound of my father's typewriter as he wrote his many books and articles.

Dr. William Timmins has been like a second father to me. He taught me the work that has become the foundation of my clinical practice, and he gave me an understanding of the underlying causes of chronic health problems.
In essence, this is his book. Dr. Timmins also taught me about integrity and the importance of listening to and learning from my patients and treating them with the respect we are all due.

Foreword

In the native societies of our ancestors, the women were extremely versatile: gathering and preparing the food, caring for the children, and protecting the home while the men were away hunting. Where they were not in obvious control of the tribe (as was the case in some Native American and various other native tribes), they exerted their influence through the men, typically allowing them to just think they were in control. Although their pivotal work among humanity is immeasurable, females are pulled by two ends of the life spectrum. They are gifted with greater connections between the left and right brain hemispheres, affording a better mix of logical and creative expression, are more neurologically efficient, and display greater intuition. But they are challenged by the fact that while Mother Nature has provided them with such a comprehensive design, She has also instilled often uncomfortable and sometimes painful physiological mechanisms to move them toward the healthiest means necessary to usher life into physical existence.

As Dr. Kalish shows you in this important and perceptive book, modern medicine has had limited success with balancing female hormones, and unfortunately has a somewhat miserable track record with all aspects of women's health, short of acute trauma intervention. Sadly, modern medicine has turned female sex organs and female hormones into a viable income stream, a virtual business endeavor — which is neither novel nor an overstatement. All the way back in 1894, William Goodell, M.D., spoke of the perils of gynecological mismanagement (1). In 1901, Byron Robinson, M.D., made the complexities and importance of caring for women correctly known to all physicians in his book Landmarks In Gynecology. In 1939, Major Bertrand DeJarnette made it clear that neither Dr. Goodell nor Dr. Robinson had been heard. In his book Bloodless Surgery, he writes:

In the treatment of diseases of women at the present time there seems to me to be a tendency to lay too much stress upon lesions of the reproductive organs. Too little heed is therefore given to the nerve-element, and, as a natural sequence, the surgical antennae of the medical profession, always too keenly sensitive, vibrate most vehemently at the approach of an ailing woman. This trend of the profession to appeal to the knife as the great panacea for woman's diseases is seen everywhere. It prevails alike in city, town, village and hamlet. It asserts itself in every medical journal. This, in my opinion, is the great medical error of the nineteenth century. It has been eloquently scored by Professor Parvin in his presidential address before the American Gynecological Society. 'There is a glamor', he says, 'about successful surgery—a flashing of swift fame, a glitter of gold and promise of financial felicity, as well as the conscious pride of success and of instant relief that may mislead, operations being done that might have been averted by judicious hygiene, and patient, wise medical treatment. It is useless to deny that unnecessary operations, sometimes sexual mutilations, are done and that many women are saved from them by changing their professional advisor.'

This commentary by the long deceased, yet still famous Dr. DeJarnette was published some 66 years ago and carries validity worthy of immediate notice to both physicians and their female patients today. Women reading this book may rest assured that the gynecological organs, female menstrual cycle, and related hormones are not Mother Nature's cruel ruse. They may also rest assured that Dr. Kalish has a proven track record of restoring health and vitality to women of all ages through natural, non-invasive means.

In this much-needed and long-overdue book, Dr. Kalish shows you how body systems co-depend on each other. For example, you will learn how key hormones, such as the stress hormone cortisol, serve as an indicator of stress perceptions produced by the interface between your external environment and internal environment. Regardless of the origin of the stress, the female body reacts predictably, utilizing vital internal resources to keep it running as close to Mother Nature's dictates as possible. While you may not find comfort in hot flashes, changes in the quality of your tissues and energy levels, it is important for you to realize that in native societies where women ate whole-food diets native to their genetic heritage (without restriction), participated in adequate exercise and were not unnecessarily poisoned by their environment, they had little, if any, discomfort with menstruation or menopause. They also gave birth easily and were often back to work contributing to family and tribal duties the next day.

I'm delighted to inform you that by following the advice offered by Dr. Kalish in Your Guide to Healthy Hormones, you stand an excellent chance of regaining the vitality now thought to have existed only among native women, while maintaining the freedoms of body, mind and spirit that every modern woman wants and well deserves!

Paul Chek
H.H.P., N.M.T.
Founder, CHEK Institute

Preface

Several years ago, a new patient came in for her initial consultation. She sat down across from me and glared. Most new patients are friendly and engaging, so I was caught off guard by her challenging attitude. She simply said, "I'm fat, I'm fatigued all the time, and I'm stressed." Then she was silent and gave me a defiant "So what are you going to do about it?" look.

In the awkward moments that followed as I struggled to formulate a response, her clear and honest appraisal of her situation led me to an epiphany. She had boldly summed up the complaints of most of my patients experiencing female hormone problems. Fat, fatigued, and stressed; overweight, overtired, and overstressed — the theme kept running through my head as a succinct description of the effects of female hormone imbalances.

For over ten years, with more than 7,000 patients, I have used natural treatments to alleviate these symptoms with noninvasive laboratory testing, natural supplements, and a focus on diet and lifestyle changes.

It is not necessary for women to become fat, fatigued, and stressed when their hormones change. Nor is it mandatory for them to take potentially harmful synthetic hormone replacement therapies. There are natural remedies available, and the goal of this book is to educate women about these safe and effective options.

And yes, that new patient who was so willing to portray her condition with painful honesty is now, years later, slim, energetic, and happy with herself again, thanks to simple changes in diet, the right kind of exercise, and an individualized nutritional supplement program. As we have come to know each other over the years, she has become a favorite patient of mine, a true inspiration to me in terms of what can be achieved using natural treatments to restore physical and emotional health.

Introduction ✖

In early 2004, millions of American women were sent into a panic. A major study on hormone replacement therapy (HRT) sponsored by a branch of the esteemed National Institutes of Health had been stopped in its tracks. The reason: Hormone replacement, long believed to help protect post-menopausal women from heart disease, not only failed to offer this protection but actually increased the risk of stroke.

The results of the Women's Health Initiative study came as dire news for some 10 million women taking hormone therapy to alleviate the symptoms of menopause and prevent disease. Worse, most of their doctors were at a loss as to what to recommend. Many women abruptly stopped taking their hormones, often prompting a recurrence of unpleasant or even incapacitating symptoms. Others reduced their dosage or switched to a hormone combination that may have been associated with other risks. (A study of a combined estrogen-progesterone drug had been cut short in 2002 when it showed an increased risk of breast cancer, heart attacks, blood clots, and strokes.)

Few women are aware that a good alternative to HRT exists. This book offers answers for the many women and medical professionals who are in a quandary about how to deal with the changes that occur in the years surrounding menopause.

I have been treating menopausal and perimenopausal women using natural therapies for twelve years. My approach is unique, in that it takes into account the underlying causes of female hormone imbalances rather than just treating symptoms. Despite what we have been led to believe, the ovaries do not spontaneously malfunction on their own; they respond to changes in other systems in the body, such as other hormones, the digestive system, and the body's detoxification system. A breakdown in hormonal function reflects a failure in how the body is handling stress and in how well the other organ systems are functioning.

Menopause is a natural phase in a complex physiological system, and each woman's body and health history is unique. There can be no single pill to treat the discomforts of menopause, yet women have been popping pills such as Premarin for the past four decades in the hope that they will offer a quick, easy solution. Now that these medications have been shown to pose a threat to health, it's time to look in a new direction.

Eastern medicine generally takes a more holistic view of the body and health, treating physical symptoms as signals from a complex, interconnected system rather than as isolated malfunctions. Western medicine is finally recognizing the wisdom of this approach, and starting to acknowledge that when part of a system breaks down, it is signaling an imbalance of the whole. It is incumbent upon the doctor to address the causes of imbalance rather than hunt for a one-size-fits-all medication aimed at treating symptoms alone.

I cannot overstate the importance of understanding menopause and responding to it in a sane way — by using safe natural treatments. More than 40 million American women are post-menopausal, and with the baby-boom generation in middle age, that number is projected to reach 60 million by 2010. So it is not just a matter of making hot flashes disappear, but of helping millions of women prevent heart disease, stroke, cancer, brittle bones, and a host of other debilitating disorders. It is a matter of restoring balance to bodies as they age, so that post-menopausal women, present and future, can enjoy the best possible quality of life.

This book aims to reverse the trend of treating a natural life process as a form of illness by examining the body's ability to heal itself.

In **Chapter One** I discuss the body's three main systems, which work in concert to keep us functioning well. I demonstrate how a breakdown in one system can cause symptoms in another, underlining the importance of restoring harmony throughout the body by addressing all three systems simultaneously.

In **Chapter Two** I examine the conventional medical approach to menopause, and why it has failed. While the standard pharmaceutical approach may succeed in controlling symptoms in a limited way, the powerful synthetic hormones used to treat menopausal women have proved too dangerous to be used.

Chapter Three looks at the functioning of two powerful hormones, estrogen and progesterone. When the three major body systems are in balance, these hormones contribute to a healthy sex drive, fat-burning ability, mental functioning, and the ability to relax the mind, sleep well, and release muscle tension. It is normal for levels of these hormones to start dropping in the years leading up to menopause, but the process can generate hormonal havoc for women with imbalances in the three major body systems, giving rise to much of the discomfort associated with menopause.

Chapter Four points out that it is, in fact, the adrenal hormones — the ones that respond to stress — that underlie most female hormone imbalances. Testing for and correcting these imbalances is crucial to addressing adrenal "burnout" and balancing the hormonal system.

Chapter Five shows how improving diet, getting appropriate exercise, and reducing stress can help restore hormonal health. I discuss the lab-based supplement programs I design to address individual women's needs.

The topic of **Chapter Six** is the little-known role of gluten sensitivity, which generates female hormone imbalance for as much as 30 percent of the U.S. population. Here I stress the importance of a change in diet for gluten-sensitive women.

Chapter Seven treats the issues of food addiction and blood sugar control. You will learn how hormone imbalances — not to mention diabetes, cancer, heart disease, and depression — are tied to obesity and blood-sugar instability.

We live in a culture in which most people are overweight and compulsively overeating. Food is an emotionally charged issue for many women, and eating disorders must be addressed in any discussion of hormone imbalance.

Chapter Eight discusses digestive tract infections, suffered unknowingly by many women who have vague symptoms such as gas, indigestion, bloating, or food cravings. Such problems are often diagnosed as irritable bowel syndrome or treated with medication to reduce stomach acid. Left untreated, these digestive problems generate hormonal disturbances that can greatly exacerbate the symptoms of menopause.

I hope this book will benefit women who are looking for ways to relieve the discomforts of menopause and other hormonal imbalances while protecting their future health. Understanding how the symptoms you are experiencing fit within your overall health will point you toward a lifestyle that optimizes your physical, mental, and emotional well-being. *Your Guide to Healthy Hormones* not only offers a road map to menopause and hormonal sanity, but starts your journey toward optimum functioning in every area of your life.

Table of Contents

Part I

Chapter 1   **The Systems Approach to Natural Healing**   1

Chapter 2   **The Medical Approach and Why It has Failed**   11

Chapter 3   **Estrogen & Progesterone:**
                    Two Key Female Hormones   19

Chapter 4   **The Adrenal Hormones**   28

Chapter 5   **The Kalish Solution to Healthy Hormones**   39

Chapter 6   **Gluten Sensitivity and Female Hormones**   56

Chapter 7   **Food Addiction and Eating Disorders**   69

Chapter 8   **Chronic Digestive System Disorders**   83

Part II   **The Kalish Diet**   94

Appendix   106

Index   111

Chapter One

The Systems Approach to Natural Healing

Emily came to my office with a host of complaints: anxiety, insomnia, decreased sex drive, low energy and stamina, neck and shoulder tension, and the early signs of osteoporosis. She was concerned about what seemed to be a steady decline in her overall health, particularly fatigue after what used to be energizing workouts. A 46-year-old mother of two, she was showing symptoms of perimenopause, the several-year stage leading up to menopause in which women typically experience a drop in certain hormone levels and some early symptoms of menopause.

Post-workout fatigue is a key indicator of problems with stress hormones, so I ran blood and saliva tests to gauge Emily's levels of estrogen, progesterone, testosterone, cortisol, DHEA (dehydroepiandosterone), and melatonin. Her estrogen levels turned out to be borderline low, and her progesterone levels were extremely low. Emily's symptoms resulted from the abnormal ratio between these hormones. She also had low levels of the stress hormones cortisol and DHEA – common among women who have experienced high stress for extended periods of time.

I treated Emily with bio-identical (plant-based) natural progesterone in a dosage that would correct her imbalance. But I could see that hormone therapy alone would not restore her health, so I prescribed a complete nutritional, dietary, and exercise program to address Emily's adrenal exhaustion.

Within three nights of starting the program, Emily's sleep and anxiety had improved. Within a month, her sex drive and energy had returned, and her neck and shoulder pain were gone. But her symptoms began to recur in the second and third months as she let her lifestyle and dietary changes lapse after the dramatic early changes – a common reaction in a culture that demands instant, permanent solutions. Maintaining good health is a daily process requiring an ongoing commitment to positive change.

Once she understood the importance of the lifestyle component of the program, Emily returned to her food regimen and earlier bedtime — a surprisingly important part of any successful hormone-balancing program. By the end of the third month, she was symptom-free. She remains so a year into her program, and will continue to do so as long as she sticks to her new food choices and daily exercise.

The Menopausal Transition

Most women experience gradual changes in their menstrual cycle between the ages of 45 and 55 before periods stop completely. During the transitional years of perimenopause, follicle production in the ovaries drops precipitously. Of the 1 million to 2 million follicles a female has in her ovaries at birth, the reserve has fallen to about a thousand by age 51, the median age for the last menstrual period. In the half year before, estrogen production also shows a steep decline, bringing on many of the symptoms of menopause and associated increase in risk for osteoporosis, heart disease, and breast and endometrial cancers.

Although each woman experiences this phase differently, many report hot flashes, insomnia, depression, fatigue, mood swings, decreased vaginal lubrication, and increased incidence of urinary tract infections, depressed sex drive, and weight gain. The hot flash, described as the sensation of heat accompanied by sweating, flushing, and chills most commonly associated with menopause, affects about 75 percent of American women for an average of four years. This nighttime discomfort often produces anxiety and insomnia, which is frequently what prompts menopausal women to seek medical help. Falling estrogen levels stimulate a rise in the stress hormone cortisol, which accelerates bone loss, disrupts sleep, and gives rise to many other symptoms.

The same dynamic can affect younger women not yet in perimenopause when adrenal exhaustion brought on by prolonged stress upsets the hormonal balance, leading to symptoms such as decreased sex drive, weight gain, fatigue, and irritability. Hormone imbalance also can manifest as premenstrual syndrome in younger, premenopausal women, with menstrual cramping, sugar cravings, hair loss, and sudden changes in mood.

The Three Body Systems

Symptoms such as Emily experienced point to an important principle in dealing with hormone imbalance: There is no simple, single solution for every situation. The hormonal system is tied in to the body's digestive and detoxification systems, and symptoms in one frequently reflect an imbalance in another. Most female hormone problems are brought on by years of poor lifestyle choices combined with digestive or detoxification issues, and in some cases the problems are complicated by a breakdown in hormone-mediated immune function that manifests as chronic sinus infections, vaginal yeast infections, or low-grade digestive tract infections.

The Hormonal System

Most signs of female hormone imbalance – including PMS and menopausal discomfort – can be traced to the adrenal, or stress, hormones that form the basis of female hormone production. During menopause, as ovarian hormone levels drop, the adrenal glands play an even greater role in maintaining hormone balance, so adrenal hormone function is the first place we look for the underlying causes of menopausal symptoms.

The adrenal hormone cortisol, best known for its pivotal role in responding to stress, also promotes the burning of body fat, helps regulate emotions, interacts with the ovarian hormones, and counters inflammation and allergies — all part of the body's "fight or flight" response to threat. Cortisol levels rise under stress, but if stress continues without enough rest for recovery — as often happens with our modern pace of life — the adrenal glands become exhausted, and cortisol levels drop. This has a chain-reaction impact on other hormones.

Estrogen is the hormone that receives the most attention in treating female hormone problems. Often referred to as the female sex hormone, it regulates the menstrual cycle and stimulates cell growth in preparation for pregnancy. Equally important is progesterone, whose diverse functions include protecting against the undesirable effects of estrogen. Progesterone helps maintain sex drive, regulate sleep, prevent anxiety, and burn body fat.

Until recent studies revealed their danger, most doctors prescribed combinations of synthetic estrogen and progesterone, or synthetic estrogen alone, to try to restore the balance of these two hormones in menopausal women. The hormones were often prescribed in high doses. In fact, Premarin, one of the most popular synthetic hormone replacements, comes in only two dosages: 0.625 milligrams and 1.25 milligrams. Just as one dress size won't fit most women, neither will one dosage.

Paula was experiencing hot flashes, night sweats, and lethargy in her mid-50s, for which her doctor prescribed a very high dosage of synthetic estrogen. Not only did that fail to relieve her symptoms, it contributed unwanted side effects (not to mention heightening her risk for developing serious illnesses down the road). Paula came to my clinic when she learned that I was successful in using natural therapies, and made the transition to a lifestyle-based natural program within a year. Today she feels that she has regained control of her life. Her mood has improved, her energy is high, and she has been able to resume a vigorous exercise program.

Natural therapies offer multiple benefits over synthetic HRT: They are safer and more effective, have fewer side effects, and can be adjusted more easily to fit a patient's needs. But they do not match the ease of taking a pill. Any natural program must be incorporated into a healthful lifestyle to work. Since hormones affect, and are affected by, the body's other major systems, all must work in concert to promote good health.

The Digestive System

The digestive system is referred to as the "mother" system because it feeds our body tissues with the nutrients we need to function. Overeating carbohydrates and sweets, poor digestive function, digestive tract infections, and food sensitivities all play a part in throwing the hormonal system off balance. Moreover, nutrition is an important first step in any hormone-rebalancing program, as your body needs key vitamins, minerals, and fatty acids to produce sex hormones. The digestive tract also must work well to properly use all the building blocks for hormonal repair. In a majority of women I have treated over the years, hormone problems have been connected to a problem in the digestive system.

The recent trend toward low-fat diets has contributed to hormone problems by reducing the building blocks (fat or cholesterol) used to produce all sex hormones, including estrogen and progesterone. People on low-fat diets often develop a lack in the fats needed to produce sex hormones. Also, for the many women who have undiagnosed sensitivities to frequently consumed foods such as grains and soy, what seems to be a healthy diet can contribute to hormone imbalance. Various dietary stresses are often a large contributor to female hormonal imbalance. Consuming the wrong foods, overeating, skipping meals, and other food-related issues such as obesity will trigger a negative hormonal response. The connection between diet and female hormones is brokered by cortisol, the stress hormone that helps to stabilize blood sugar. If you eat a lot of sweets or refined grains, your blood sugar level becomes unstable, forcing your body to restabilize these levels by producing insulin and — eventually — large amounts of cortisol. Giving in to a craving for sweets at times of stress only feeds a vicious cycle: The sugar throws your hormones out of balance, raising stress levels, giving rise to a craving for sweets. Over time, these fluctuations in cortisol have a profound impact on the sex hormones.

The typical American diet only encourages such an imbalance. We tend to start the day with sugary, high-starch foods such as muffins and sweetened cereal without balancing these carbohydrates with sufficient protein or healthy fat. Adding even a small amount of protein to such a meal can cut insulin levels by half, helping to balance hormone levels. Since each hormone can affect another, changes in progesterone levels can affect insulin; insulin can affect cortisol, and so on. Our hormones act as a constant emergency response team, responding to triggers ranging from excessive intake of sugar and caffeine to constant worrying. Hormones rarely cause problems on their own. In most cases, they react to various types of stress. If we can identify and remove the stress causing the hormone imbalance, the correction is viable to last.

Food allergies are another important digestive factor affecting daily and monthly hormone cycles. Sensitivity to gluten (found in many grains) is the most common food reaction triggering hormone imbalance, yet it often goes undiagnosed or misdiagnosed. Those at highest risk are of Northern and Eastern European heritage. If untreated, gluten intolerance can bring low energy, depression, obesity, and diabetes as well as very high rates of osteoporosis.

Food sensitivities to soy or pasteurized dairy products are yet another common problem with the digestive system that I see among menopausal women, especially since soy has been promoted as helping to balance hormone levels and is widely used by women experiencing hormone problems. Many women who are adding large amounts of soy to their diets are unknowingly allergic to it. While soy can benefit some women in Asian cultures, it is traditionally eaten as a small part of their diet, in combination with foods that balance out its nutrient profile, and prepared in ways that aid its digestion. Soy causes problems for many women in the form of protein powders, protein bars, and other processed food items.

Problems with the digestive system are the most common underlying cause of hormone imbalance in the patients I have treated. In a minority of cases, I have found the underlying cause to be with the body's third major system, the detoxification system.

The Detoxification System

Detoxification pathways remove harmful chemicals generated from normal body functions such as physical exertion and breathing, which generate waste products that also need to be removed from the tissues. Detoxification pathways are also busy removing alcohol and metabolizing (breaking down) medications, chemicals in our food such as pesticides and herbicides, along with pollution we are exposed to in our air and water. If you are taking in more toxins than you can flush out through the liver, kidneys, stool, and skin, you will have a backlog of waste products in the body that can cause a large number of symptoms. If the liver detoxification pathways are unable to handle their burden, you will have trouble metabolizing (breaking down) hormones — a problem commonly seen among women who respond poorly to synthetic hormones.

Consumption of alcohol, sugar, medications, and synthetic hormones over the course of a woman's life all contribute to clogging the liver detoxification pathways, which are alternately helped by eating healthful sources of protein and vegetables. Vegetarians who eat insufficient protein are at risk for detox problems, as are women who have not eaten sufficient vegetables. Liver detox pathways can be corrected through both diet and supplements.

Improving the Three Systems

All three body systems— hormonal, digestive, and detoxification— can be improved through simple changes in lifestyle and diet. In some cases, these lifestyle changes are enough to resolve problems; in others, nutritional supplements are necessary. In cases where multiple problems may have been brewing for years, lab testing may be needed to pinpoint causes so that a customized therapeutic diet and supplement program can be designed.

It certainly takes some detective work to diagnose the causes of each woman's symptoms and determine the best course of treatment, and it takes determination on the woman's part to stay with a program and maintain it for the long term. But what better reward is there than good health?

Chapter Two
The Medical Approach and Why It has Failed

Menopause is a natural transition ending the body's childbearing phase, and has been around for as long as women have. But it has not caused women at all times and in all places the kinds of complications we associate with it today. In the West, menopause was simply not talked about in polite company — until recently. Alarm over the dangers of hormone replacement therapy have brought the topic out in the open, and cast a sharp light on the medical establishment's abysmal failure to address an issue that all women will encounter in midlife.

The conventional Western view of the female reproductive system becomes evident from the vocabulary used to describe it. The essential female hormone estrogen derives from the Greek estrus, meaning "frenzy." The Greek word for uterus, hystera, forms the root for hysterical. Little has changed in terms of linking "female trouble" with insanity over the centuries: The current medical model typically ties menopause to depression, and responds by prescribing antidepressants.

In 1966 the first highly influential book appeared on the use of synthetic hormone replacement therapy (HRT), Feminine Forever. Its author, Dr. Ronald Wilson, had his research and book paid for by Wyeth, the pharmaceutical company that manufactures the drug Premarin. A prominent gynecologist, Wilson received funding to start a research organization that legitimized the use of hormones for treating problems associated with menopause.

Wilson's attitude toward menopause represented no great leap forward. In Feminine Forever, he describes menopause as a "living decay" in which women descend to a "vapid cow-like state." His best-selling book promoted Premarin as a panacea for this deplorable fate, and Wyeth ignored the questionable methods used in Wilson's research.

By the early 1970s, the synthetic estrogen supplement Premarin had become the all-purpose treatment for menopause, and it continued to be prescribed widely for the next 30 years, despite a study in 1975 that linked estrogen replacement therapy (ERT) to uterine cancer. This finding stalled the ERT bandwagon only briefly. Adding progestins to the mix — synthetic progesterone — resulted in a drug that was considered safer, and ERT became the more comprehensive hormone replacement therapy that is still used by millions of women in this country.

Two Disturbing Studies

It wasn't until July 2001 that the risks of synthetic hormone replacement became widely known. An eight-year government-funded study of more than 16,000 American women by the Women's Health Initiative showed that Prempro — the synthetic hormones Premarin plus Provera — were shown to increase the risk of breast cancer by 26 percent, heart attacks by 29 percent, and stroke by 41 percent, while more than doubling the risk of blood clots and pulmonary embolisms. Prempro was shown to reduce colon cancer and promote bone density. But elevated death rates from heart attacks, stroke, pulmonary embolisms, and breast cancer were so alarming that researchers halted the study three years early, saying it was too dangerous to allow the research subjects to continue taking the drug combination.

The effects of this study were far-reaching. In the year it was published, U.S. pharmacists filled some 45 million prescriptions for Premarin and 22 million for Prempro, and an estimated 38 percent of American women were on synthetic HRT. Tens of millions of menopausal women didn't know where to turn. Many weighed the risks and remained on synthetic hormones. And doctors continued prescribing the drugs for short-term use, reasoning that the study had focused on long-term effects.

The role of doctors in the hormone-replacement controversy remains unclear. Dr. Susan Love, author of Dr. Susan Love's Menopause and Hormone Book, is a prominent women's health specialist and long-time critic of HRT. She charges, "The incestuous relationship between the pharmaceutical companies and the medical establishment is part of it. A lot of information doctors get is channeled through the drug companies."[2] The American College of Obstetrics and Gynecology, responding to the study findings, created a task force to rethink its guidelines on HRT. The task force chairman, Dr. Isaac Schiff of Massachusetts General Hospital, declared: "Ten years ago it was almost malpractice not to endorse estrogen. Now the bubble has burst."[3]

If nothing else, doctors had failed to question the safety of synthetic hormones, ignoring earlier studies that pointed to a problem. It took concerned women in positions of power to push the medical establishment to take up the issue. The Women's Health Initiative, launched in 1991 by women's groups and female legislators including outspoken U.S. Rep. Pat Schroeder, took several more years to get research funding. Schroeder, the former Democratic congresswoman from Colorado, fumed that in the late 1970s the largest study conducted by the National Institute on Aging hadn't included a single woman. "They didn't know anything about osteoporosis, menopause, anything," she told Time. "They wouldn't do anything for women but throw pills at them."[4]

Change happens slowly in the medical establishment. After the initial alarm over the dangers of HRT, public concern faded with the headlines. It took another study, this time of estrogen alone, to drive the point home. The study was again conducted by the Women's Health Initiative and again aborted when researchers found that estrogen not only failed to reduce the risk of coronary heart disease, it increased the risk of stroke.

Another wave of women discontinued their therapy. Prescriptions for hormone replacement drugs plummeted during the twelve months following the release of the study. According to the Journal of the American Medical Association, sales of HRT drugs fell 38 percent; sales of Prempro, the popular estrogen-progesterone cocktail that was the subject of the first WHI study, fell 74 percent, as stated in June 2004 in the New York Times. Research commissioned by drug companies showed that 18.5 million American women were using HRT in 2002, and only 7.6 million by January 2004. Women who continued to take synthetic hormones to treat menopause did so uneasily, feeling they had no alternative. But a large number of women, skeptical of the medical establishment's sincere concern for their well-being, undertook research on their own. Some of these women eventually end up in my office seeking a more holistic approach to their health.

Meanwhile, the cycle continues. The New York Times article also states that recent studies show the drop in HRT use is bottoming out, and some doctors are seeing increased demand for synthetic hormones. Eager to meet the demand, drug manufacturers are offering lower-dose versions that are widely presumed (though not proven) to be safer. Dr. JoAnn E. Manson, chief of preventive medicine at Harvard University's Brigham and Women's Hospital in Boston and a principal investigator for the Women's Health Initiative, offered this precaution: "Until proven otherwise, we should assume all medications in a similar class have similar risk. It's biologically plausible that a lower dose might have a lower risk, but we don't know yet."[5] Given the number of years it takes to complete a well-designed study, millions of women may be jeopardizing their health awaiting the results.

Synthetic Estrogen: The Quick Fix

Just like the women who want a pill to dissolve their menopausal problems, researchers and the drug companies that fund their work ache for a simple solution. That's why they have focused for so long on estrogen: It has been known for decades that depletion of this hormone plays an essential role in the effects of menopause. It turns out, however, that estrogen imbalances can't be resolved simply by adding estrogen. The issue is much more complex.

The various sex and stress hormones — including estrogen, progesterone, testosterone, cortisol, and DHEA — function in relation to one another in a balance known as homeostasis. A drop in estrogen will trigger a rise in cortisol; a rise in cortisol will first raise and then eventually trigger a drop in DHEA, and so on in a process that favors equilibrium. Under conditions of prolonged stress, for example, the body reacts by diverting hormone production from sex hormones to stress hormones. This is a built-in survival mechanism: Under extreme stress, sex hormone production becomes a luxury we can do without.

The quick-fix treatment for menopause ignores this relationship. Researchers chose the most powerful sex hormone and concentrated it into a toxic dose that worked the magic of alleviating menopausal symptoms for many women, and filled the coffers of drug companies and their investors. The drug's long-term consequences were underestimated or ignored. Moreover, the one-size-fits-all approach resulted in highly concentrated doses of Premarin that are eight to ten times what most women need.[6] It was easier, after all, for the manufacturers and medical establishment to create a few standard sizes to fit all bodies rather than determine what individual patients need — just as some clothing manufacturers cut corners by offering the ill-fitting approach of small, medium, and large.

There is a fragile balance between the essential female hormones estrogen and progesterone, which are supplemented in hormone replacement therapy. It is virtually impossible to achieve a healthy natural balance for any individual woman using the drugs available. Even if a drug alleviates symptoms, it does nothing to address the imbalance causing them, which eventually will lead to problems systemwide. What appears to us as a malfunction or symptom is usually a response to disruption in the normal production of hormones. For example, you might be using up progesterone in response to emotional or dietary stress or hidden inflammation, upsetting the estrogen-progesterone balance. Simply adding synthetic progesterone — the conventional solution — may mask the problem but will do nothing to address the underlying issue. The only truly effective treatment is to assess and correct the major sources of stress and the hormonal response to it, using safer, nature-based products in conjunction with lifestyle changes.

Looking to the Future

While the conventional scientific approach has failed menopausal women, it has succeeded in calling attention to its own dangers. Negative publicity surrounding HRT has been a wake-up call leading women to search for alternatives and demand changes from the medical establishment. As a result, more doctors are turning their attention to safer, effective treatments for their patients. And these treatments do exist.

The following chapters will examine an alternative approach, not only to solving a problem, but also to achieving physical, mental, and emotional health. My patients have truly been my teachers, and they have made it clear to me that treating symptoms while ignoring their causes is inherently dangerous. I'll explain how my technique, combining scientific testing and natural treatment, can safely restore imbalances and put women on the track to health.

Notes

1. Christine Gorman and Alice Park, "The Truth About Hormones." Time, July 22, 2002.

2. Geoffrey Cowley and Karen Springen, "The End of the Age of Estrogen." Newsweek, July 22, 2002.

3. Gorman and Park.

4. Gorman and Park.

5. Leslie Berger, "On Hormone Therapy, the Dust Is Still Settling." The New York Times, June 6, 2004, section 15, p. 10.

6. Cohen, Jay S. Overdose: The Case Against the Drug Companies: Prescription Drugs, Side Effects and Your Health. New York: Jeremy P. Tarcher / Putnam, 2001.

Chapter 3
Estrogen & Progesterone:
Two Key Female Hormones

Few people had much awareness of estrogen and progesterone until recent studies revealed the dangers of female hormone replacement therapy. Millions of women had been taking synthetic hormones for years, yet the role these hormones play is still largely misunderstood. The goal of this chapter is to clear up some of the confusion.

The Role of Estrogen

While the dangers of hormone replacement therapy may have given estrogen a bad name, this vital hormone contributes greatly to a woman's health when maintained in a natural balance. Estrogen is responsible for female sexual development at puberty. As a foundation to fertility, estrogen promotes accumulation of fat in the hips, thighs, and breasts. It causes the lining of the uterus to grow and thicken every month in preparation for a fertilized egg. At the end of the menstrual cycle, this lining is shed as estrogen levels drop. Another essential role this hormone plays is to promote the movement of salt and minerals into cells.

For decades, drug companies and doctors pointed to estrogen deficiency as the main problem behind the common symptoms of menopause. For those of us who practice natural medicine, however, these same symptoms signal an imbalance in both the ovarian hormones and those that generate the stress response. We believe that the solution lies in re-establishing the natural balance of multiple hormones, rather than simply increasing the amount of estrogen in a woman's system.

Estrogen, Diet, and Exercise

Dr. Peter Ellison of Harvard University, who pioneered the use of salivary testing that I incorporate in my practice, found that women in industrialized nations have abnormally high levels of estrogen, which he links to our high levels of breast and uterine cancer. As documented in Dr. John Lee's book Natural Progesterone, the results of Dr. Ellison's studies demonstrate a relationship between hormone levels, diet, and exercise worldwide. Inactive women who consume more calories than they burn have elevated levels of estrogen, which may help explain high estrogen levels among American women, a majority of whom are overweight and obese. The natural drop in estrogen levels with the approach of menopause will be steeper in these women, leading to a corresponding rise in cortisol production. This intensifies any symptoms related to stress, and gives rise to a host of problems related to cortisol, including insomnia, hot flashes, night sweats, and mood swings. This may help explain why women in technologically advanced Western countries with higher estrogen levels report more pronounced menopausal symptoms than women in less-developed nations.

A 1998 study of 625 female runners in the United States supports Dr. Ellison's theory. The runners had higher levels of physical activity and far less obesity than average women, and reported being able to reduce the discomforts of menopause with increased exercise. Indeed, for some women, changes in diet and exercise alone can eliminate many menopausal symptoms.

Estrogen and Environmental Factors

High estrogen levels are also promoted by environmental factors. Exposure to xenoestrogens (chemical compounds widely found in our environment) exert a powerful estrogen-like effect on the female body. These toxic compounds are most commonly encountered as by-products of the petrochemical industry, and we are exposed to them during the course of many daily activities, such as when plastic or Styrofoam containers are heated in a microwave, or when we eat food wrapped in plastic or drink water from plastic bottles. The hormones added to our food supply are another source of increased estrogen levels. Many of the conveniences of modern life are contributing to hormonal imbalances in American women.

How Estrogen Affects the Body

While estrogen is needed for healthy functioning, too much of it has a negative impact on a woman's cardiovascular system. It promotes blood clots in the lungs, increases the risk of heart attack, contributes to blood vessel spasms, elevates blood pressure, and lowers the blood's oxygen-carrying capacity. It is therefore not surprising that estrogen replacement therapy, in which women are given high levels of synthetic estrogen, has been linked to an increased risk of cardiovascular disease.

Another role of estrogen is to stimulate cell growth. Therefore, when taken in excess, estrogen causes excessive cell growth and increases the risk of certain types of cancer, including breast cancer.

Excess estrogen is also associated with other health problems that, while less dangerous, are uncomfortable and potentially debilitating, such as the water retention that many women experience as bloating and weight gain, and an increase in gall bladder problems. It also causes a loss of zinc, a mineral vital to the repair of soft tissue. Low zinc levels make it more difficult to recover from injury and affect immune function, making people more susceptible to colds and flu.

The Role of Progesterone

Chronic stress reduces progesterone levels, and affects the levels of two other important hormones, cortisol and DHEA, which are central to many body functions. Our modern diet is also responsible for lowering progesterone levels. Our increasing reliance on grains and decreased consumption of fruits and vegetables contribute to this trend.

The Estrogen-Progesterone Balance

In most of my patients I have tested, low progesterone levels are exacerbating the effects of estrogen imbalances. It is the correct balance between these two hormones that maintains healthy functioning, while an imbalance can lead to a range of problems. In some women, low estrogen triggers the imbalance. Estrogen levels normally decline with age, but if stress hormones remain balanced, few symptoms occur. However, women as young as 30 can experience prematurely low estrogen levels, leading to low sex drive, infertility, dry or wrinkled skin, excess fat deposition (especially around the waist and back of the thighs), inability to lose weight despite dieting and exercise, and migraine headaches. Depending on each individual patient's estrogen levels, treatment options must be configured differently.

Also, many women have more than one factor contributing to hormone imbalance, such as low estrogen combined with low progesterone and high stress hormone levels. It is hardly surprising that they exhibit symptoms ranging from mood swings to insomnia. Estrogen-progesterone imbalances are not exclusive to menopausal women.

In menstruating women, estrogen peaks at ovulation, around two weeks into the typical 28-day cycle. This is followed by a surge of progesterone in the second half of the cycle as the egg is released. This natural cycle can be disrupted, however, by disturbances in the circadian rhythm, or 24-hour cycle, of production of the essential hormone cortisol. The daily rhythm is the driving force behind regulating the monthly cycle, and when cortisol levels are disturbed by irregular sleep patterns, skipped meals, emotional stress, or other factors, the result is hormonal symptoms. In effect, the entire system becomes imbalanced.

Correcting Hormonal Imbalance

In the majority of my patients, sex hormone symptoms can be eliminated by making certain lifestyle changes and by balancing adrenal hormones. As we will see in the next chapter, high levels of these stress hormones often cause or worsen many menopausal symptoms. Women with imbalances of the stress hormones cortisol and DHEA often develop problems at menopause, when the ovaries rely more heavily on estrogen produced by the adrenal glands. Under chronic stress, demand rises for cortisol and DHEA at the expense of producing progesterone. This effect is intensified by the rise in cortisol triggered by the normal drop in estrogen at midlife. At this stage of life, many women will require the support of natural, or bio-identical, progesterone.

Progesterone creams have become popular because they can be bought without a prescription. They are fast-acting because they are absorbed directly and rapidly into the bloodstream. However, it is difficult to get exact dosages each day, and some women build up high progesterone levels with extended use. High progesterone levels can lead to symptoms such as fatigue, insomnia, and depression. Furthermore, some women have an enzyme that converts progesterone from the creams into other hormone compounds, and this can interfere with successful treatment.

Bio-identical progesterone taken under the tongue in liquid form tends to be the best option for most women. It's easiest to get precise daily doses, and like creams these forms deliver hormones directly to the bloodstream.

Likewise, many women who are low in estrogen require the use of bio-identical estrogen to achieve hormone balance. Natural estrogen can be prescribed in pills, gels, patches, or troches (sublingual lozenges). When a patient chooses one of these forms of prescription estrogen, I work with her medical doctor to coordinate this treatment with the rest of her program. Patients also can use phytoestrogen compounds — natural, plant-based formulas — that can be obtained without a prescription. I have found that most of my patients who are willing to improve their diet and exercise patterns will have complete symptom relief by using an adrenal hormone program plus plant-based natural progesterone and estrogen.

Insulin is yet another hormone we produce that coordinates with our sex and stress hormones. Patients with a condition known variously as Metabolic Syndrome, Syndrome X, or insulin resistance will not fully benefit from the typical female hormone programs until their metabolism is healed. Dr. Diana Schwarzbein, an endocrinologist in Santa Barbara, California, who has used bio-identical hormone programs with thousands of patients, has pioneered the use of bio-identical female hormone therapy in conjunction with lifestyle changes. Her books are a must-read for anyone who wants to learn more about this subject.

Progesterone Testimonial

Dr. Kalish: One of my patients provides a prime example of estrogen-progesterone imbalance. Helen is a 58-year-old athlete with a long history of hormonal problems that led her to undergo a hysterectomy followed by hormone replacement.

Helen: When I went to Dr. Kalish, I was desperate and — to be honest — quite pessimistic. An athlete friend of mine who is a long-standing patient of his suggested I go when I complained to her about my inability to lose weight even though I was eating healthy and exercising several times a week. She said that he did natural hormone replacement therapy, and this intrigued me because I've always been interested in natural health alternatives and I wasn't feeling any better with the hormone replacement therapy I was prescribed after my hysterectomy.

Dr. Kalish: When I first saw Helen, she was frustrated by her inability to lose weight despite a restricted diet and a heavy training schedule. She was experiencing back and lower-extremity joint pain after running. She also reluctantly admitted to feeling moody and depressed after starting an estrogen regimen, and her symptoms were getting worse.

Helen: I had a good feeling about Dr. Kalish right off the bat. The first thing he did was reassure me that my problems were normal and that he had successfully treated thousands of women just like me! This was hopeful news, and I was excited to find out the results of the lab tests that he ordered for me.

Dr. Kalish: Lab testing showed that Helen's estrogen levels while using HRT were alarmingly high. Since she wasn't taking any progesterone, her ratio of progesterone to estrogen was greatly disturbed. She needed to lower her estrogen dosage and increase her progesterone levels.

Helen: When Dr. Kalish explained my lab results to me in my follow-up consultation, I was shocked and somewhat angry that I had been prescribed such an excessive dosage of estrogen. I was very curious to see the results of Dr. Kalish's treatment.

Dr. Kalish: After only a few weeks of treatment with bio-identical progesterone, and a shift to a bio-identical estrogen at the appropriate dosage, Helen's mood swings were gone and her depression had greatly diminished. Without the excess water weight and body fat promoted by the estrogen, she returned to her normal weight. The progesterone also had an anti-inflammatory effect, helping her to resume her running program without the constant joint pain.

Helen: It's been six months, and I am feeling much more like myself these days. I am able to maintain my weight, and the occasional migraines I was having have vanished. I have been given my vitality back, and I am living the kind of active life I love.

Unfortunately, Helen's situation is far from unusual. In addition to placing themselves at heightened risk of life-threatening illnesses, many women on HRT are only disturbing further their estrogen-progesterone ratio. My technique of carefully testing hormone levels, combined with a more healthful diet, adequate exercise, and stress reduction, can put their lives back on track.

Chapter Four
The Adrenal Hormones

While most publicity on hormones has focused on estrogen and progesterone, the adrenal hormones may well play the most crucial role in female hormone imbalance. These hormones, including cortisol and DHEA, are secreted by a pair of ductless glands above the kidneys in response to stress. When women experience too much stress for too long, the ovarian hormones are eventually affected. In fact, it is commonly the stress response that triggers female hormone imbalance and its symptoms.

The Role of Cortisol

Cortisol, one of several hormones produced by the adrenal glands, plays a pivotal role in the hormonal system. Cortisol helps regulate blood pressure and cardiovascular function, as well as the metabolism of proteins, carbohydrates, and fats. Cortisol is secreted in response to any stress in the body, physical or psychological, leading to a breakdown of muscle protein, which releases amino acids into the bloodstream that are then converted by the liver into energy. Cortisol also mobilizes glycogen (stored glucose or sugar) from the liver to generate energy.

The body has an elaborate system for controlling cortisol secretion. Stress typically triggers the release of hormones that increase production of cortisol, among other hormones, to prepare the body for action and protect it from damage in the event of traumatic injury. After the stressful event has passed, the hormone levels return to normal. With chronic or repeated stress, however, the body continues to produce cortisol. If the adrenal glands are perpetually called upon to produce cortisol, they eventually weaken, leading to adrenal fatigue and ultimately exhaustion — adrenal burnout — which can increase body fat and cause fatigue and depression, among other symptoms.

Adrenal Exhaustion

With stress, a surge of cortisol prepares the body to fight off an attack or flee. For millennia this mechanism operated under conditions that would be followed by long periods of rest and full recovery. Today, however, we are essentially locked in a culture-wide "fight or flight" state. In my new patients I have found their poor diets, lack of exercise and sleep, and long work hours leave their bodies in a chronic state of stress, with many restorative functions continually sacrificed or impaired.

If elevated stress continues for months or years, higher-than-normal cortisol levels can no longer be maintained, and the hormone levels start to plummet. In laboratory tests of my patients I have repeatedly seen the first sign of adrenal exhaustion, a drop in DHEA accompanying high cortisol — a sign that other hormones are being affected. In patients who are even more stressed, I see Stage 2 of adrenal exhaustion: The once-high cortisol levels have fallen, with even lower DHEA. Finally, in Stage 3 of adrenal exhaustion, both cortisol and DHEA become dangerously low.

Most women feel good in Stage 1 of adrenal exhaustion. Although they are under stress, their cortisol levels remain high, and this provides a rush of energy as the body burns through its hormonal reserves. This state is reflective of modern American culture, in which achievement-oriented and overworked people have become the norm.

Women with genetically strong adrenal glands can carry on in Stage 1 for many years or even decades, while others crash and burn early on. Most people don't slow down until they experience some type of health problem or emotional crisis that forces them to re-evaluate their pace of living. My clinical experience has shown that this happens around the time patients move from Stage 2 (which does not feel good, but is survivable, fueled with enough caffeine and sugar) to Stage 3, when it becomes clear that something is wrong.

Stage 3 patients may be tired all the time, unable to lose weight as in the past, be depressed, or have low sex drive. As a woman progresses from Stage 1 to 3 of adrenal exhaustion, her female hormone symptoms will predictably worsen. Irregular menstrual periods, PMS, and early menopause are common among my patients experiencing a breakdown of adrenal reserves. Most women with perimenopausal or menopausal symptoms are in Stage 2 or 3 of adrenal exhaustion. A woman in Stage 3 who enters perimenopause will see what was once a couple of rough days each month turn into "menopausal madness."

Adrenal exhaustion compromises the body's ability to compensate for acute stress, leaving a person feeling lethargic, fatigued, and susceptible to chronic illness. An abnormal adrenal rhythm also impacts:

- ✤ Skin regeneration, causing wrinkles and premature aging
- ✤ Sleep quality, leading to trouble falling and staying asleep
- ✤ Bone health, which creates osteopenia, or bone loss
- ✤ Muscle and joint function, leading to achy, arthritis-type joint pain and neck, shoulder, and lower back pain
- ✤ Immune function, leading to frequent illness

In short, adrenal hormone production is an indicator of overall body function, and an imbalance in this system is a sign of chronic illness. It is therefore vital to address any adrenal malfunction in women displaying menopausal symptoms.

The Role of DHEA

Another adrenal hormone that needs to be kept in balance is dihydroepiandosterone, commonly known as DHEA. This hormone is produced through the action of the hormone pregnenolone and is also a precursor to estrogen. When we are healthy and unstressed, cortisol and DHEA levels remain stable. Deviations mean that the body is compensating for underlying stress.

When DHEA production is disturbed because of stress, there is a breakdown in its conversion to estrogen, and stress can therefore impact estrogen levels, leading to hormonal symptoms. At the same time, pregnenolone is diverted to produce cortisol, which can lower progesterone, further exacerbating the female hormone symptoms. The entire system of female hormones is thus disrupted. To make matters worse, under normal circumstances DHEA production, which peaks in a woman's mid-20s, declines steadily from her early 30s, so that the average 75-year-old has only 20 percent of the DHEA of a woman of 25. Cortisol levels, meanwhile, tend to increase with age, so women are quite likely to have a cortisol-DHEA imbalance by the time they reach menopause. In fact, it is normal to have cortisol levels rise in response to dropping estrogen levels that occur at perimenopause.

Unfortunately, as is the case with estrogen and progesterone, many women supplement with DHEA without first determining their individual needs. This potent steroidal hormone is widely available as an over-the-counter dietary supplement that has been advertised as promoting weight loss and longevity and preventing disease. But it is often taken in unregulated amounts that can lead to serious side effects. As with all hormones, DHEA should be taken only as directed by a health professional who has determined the correct dosage based on lab testing. Cortisol-boosting supplements are also popular right now, and many of my patients have tried them unsuccessfully, because they did so without adequate lab testing to determine what is required. These cortisol-related supplements help temporarily, only to lead to further problems down the road.

Adrenal Hormones and Chronic Stress

We all experience stress in our lives, much of it related to lifestyle. Many women have to juggle demanding jobs and family responsibilities, leaving them physically and emotionally exhausted by the end of the day. Others may be caring for ailing parents. Financial hardship and strained relationships also create major prolonged stress, which is complicated by health-related issues such as poor diet, irregular sleep patterns, chemical toxicity, injury, or infection. Anxiety and fear are also sources of stress, such as the recent fear of terrorism in this country. Stress is usually caused by multiple factors.

Some people are naturally better at handling stress, and have healthier adrenal hormone function as a result. But when the adrenal glands are overstressed and weakened, it is important to address the causes, possibly through further testing for undiagnosed health conditions. In most cases, some type of lifestyle modification is called for. As Americans sleep less, eat more fast food on the run, and lead more sedentary lives glued to computer screens and cell phones, their ability to handle daily stress and lead balanced lives has diminished. It's no wonder so many American women complain of the symptoms of menopause!

Stress

There are three important stages to consider with regard to stress: perception, response, and internalization. These mark the "flow" of our stress response, and the ways in which we manage and evaluate them are crucial.

When stress occurs, the first thing we do is perceive it. Next, we respond to it. Lastly, we internalize the stress. It is the internalization of stress that is key. Stress that is internalized negatively will have lasting effects. For this reason, we must find effective individual techniques for stress reduction. People are unique, and the ways they reduce stress reflects this. For some, effective stress reduction could be yoga. For others, it is running or golf. It may be meditating or gardening or keeping a journal. Many people benefit from learning about themselves through classes, books, or seeing a therapist or psychologist. Stress reduction is essential to achieving emotional and spiritual health, which will directly affect your physical health and well-being.

Adrenal Hormones and Weight Gain

Cortisol is a glucocorticosteroid hormone. This is a fancy way of saying cortisol levels shift in response to what you eat. If you eat too much sugar or too many carbohydrates, excess insulin and then excess cortisol are released, leading to increased fat storage and weight gain. Excess cortisol is thus linked to increased fat storage and obesity. Moreover, a recent study on eating disorders found that women who secreted higher levels of cortisol under stress had a greater tendency to snack on high-fat food than those who secreted less. Women who insist they can't take off excess weight during menopause often have valid reasons for their complaint, because adrenal dysfunction slows down metabolism and increases body fat. High cortisol also has been linked to low thyroid function and lowered metabolic rate — issues central to many women's menopausal concerns.

Adrenal Hormones and Mood Disorders

An overactive stress response can bring on depression, anxiety, and panic attacks, while underactivity has been associated with fatigue, lethargy, and apathy —symptoms of depression. There is a strong relationship between cortisol secretion patterns and mood fluctuations.

People suffering from depression often show a disruption in their circadian (daily) rhythm of cortisol fluctuations, resulting in abnormally high morning and midnight levels of the hormone, precipitating sleep disruption and a variety of mood disorders. Research studies have shown that as many as seven out of ten patients with depression have an enlarged adrenal gland — approximately 1.7 times larger than healthy subjects, a result of increased stress hormone production.

Many of my patients whose past treatments failed to restore proper hormonal balance have had problems metabolizing or eliminating hormones. If your liver has become damaged and inflamed by the use of alcohol, prescription drugs, or by a poor diet, then you will likely have a poor response to hormone treatments.

This type of internal-organ stress is referred to as hidden inflammation — for obvious reasons. When an internal organ is inflamed, the symptoms may mask the true underlying cause. For example, inflammation of the stomach can feel like chest pain or neck pain; intestinal inflammation can feel like low back pain.

Hidden Inflammation and Stress

An appropriate treatment plan for adrenal hormone imbalance often includes low dosages of DHEA, supplements such as pregnenolone, and minerals including magnesium and calcium. It also may include changes in diet and exercise, and various forms of stress reduction. Most of my patients have found dietary changes to be central to achieving hormone balance. Our current dieting trends tend to promote weight loss by increasing cortisol. Even though we end up thinner, we are left significantly more stressed out. Of course, when we go off the latest "diet" and eat normally, we calm down and gain back all the weight! I see this pattern every single day in my patients.

In all the thousands of women I have tested, the gastrointestinal system is the body system that most frequently suffers from chronic inflammation. This includes the stomach, small intestine, and colon. Symptoms of inflammation in the digestive organs may be vague or hard to interpret, but about half the women I've examined thoroughly have at least one undiagnosed digestive tract infection causing inflammation, which elevates cortisol and triggers female hormone problems.

Adrenal Testimonial

Dr. Kalish: Kathryn offers a classic example of adrenal burnout. When she came to see me, she was overweight, excessively fatigued and feeling very stressed. She had been having panic attacks for some time.

Kathryn: I've always been a very high-strung, controlling person. I was always the overachiever who did things better and faster. Right out of college, I got a stressful job with a prominent accounting firm. The hours were grueling, the stress unavoidable, especially for me. About three years after starting my job, I had gained a considerable amount of weight and was having frequent panic attacks. I even landed in the emergency room a few times. When I wasn't worked up about something or other at work, I was exhausted. All I ever wanted to do in my free time was sleep. I was only 25 years old. Something was wrong.

Dr. Kalish: Kathryn had been under constant stress for quite some time, and it was finally getting to her. Between the long hours she was putting in at work, her lack of exercise and poor diet, she was setting herself up for adrenal exhaustion. I explained to Kathryn that our bodies are designed to handle stress by releasing cortisol, which prepares the body to protect itself. But the body needs time to return to normal after the stressful situation is over. The problem with Kathryn and with many Americans is that she was under constant stress — her body never had time to recover. It was not surprising that under chronic stress Kathryn was experiencing weight gain, fatigue, and panic attacks. Sometimes this is referred to as feeling "wired and tired."

Kathryn: I understood what Dr. Kalish was telling me. It made sense. It also became obvious that something was seriously out of balance in my body. Dr. Kalish had me do a series of saliva tests to determine my stress hormone levels. Once we got the results back, he was able to help me determine what supplements I should take, as well as what dietary and lifestyle changes would help to lower my stress.

Dr. Kalish: Even before we had set up Kathryn with the supplements necessary to reprogram her hormones, I recommended that she follow the Kalish Solution Diet, which would eliminate gluten and emphasize protein, vegetables, non-gluten carbohydrates, and healthy fats. In addition, I recommended that she give up her customary glass or two of red wine every night, and instead drink more water.

Kathryn: Dr. Kalish's dietary suggestions were very useful. I followed them religiously, and noticed results very early on. I was experiencing less fatigue and I eventually started to lose weight. Dr. Kalish also suggested I go to a counselor to help me deal with the stress and anxiety that I had been experiencing. I now go to a counselor once a week, and find it very useful to release some of my tension. I still get stressed sometimes, but my therapist, along with my hormone treatment, have made these instances few and far between, and I now have more tools to combat the stress when it rears its ugly head.

Chapter Five
The Kalish Solution to Healthy Hormones

During my first year of clinical practice, I became fascinated by technical manuals written by the great teachers of endocrinology in alternative medicine, and began to focus on using bio-identical (natural) progesterone. In the years since, I have studied with many of the top experts in natural hormone therapies — naturopaths, medical doctors, nutritionists, biochemists, directors of medical laboratories, and chiropractors. Over the last twelve years, based on work with more than 7,000 patients, I have been able to test the various theories taught to me. The product of this work is a system of diagnosis and treatment I call the Kalish Solution.

The Kalish Solution has provided natural health solutions to thousands of my patients, and I hope this book will allow these principles to benefit a larger population. Although my practice has been oriented around female hormone programs, I have worked with patients of many other profiles, using the same model to treat fatigue, weight gain, digestive problems such as bloating, heartburn, irritable bowel syndrome; and even autoimmune conditions. The reason for my success is simple: Most chronic conditions involve problems with one or more of the body's three main systems described in Chapter 2.

Assessing and correcting the functioning of the three body systems can benefit a host of conditions by addressing their underlying causes. As a society, we have become so symptom-oriented, taking a pill for this and an herb for that, that we have lost sight of the interdependence of most body systems. Symptom in Latin means "signal," and a symptom indeed signals that one of the body systems has stopped functioning properly. If you ignore your symptoms for long enough, they worsen and may lead to disease. Even when diseases don't develop, quality of life decreases.

This is a difficult situation for most physicians to address, because they are trained to treat either symptoms or diseases. For example, if a patient has hot flashes — a symptom involving a complex array of hormone fluctuations — most doctors prescribe estrogen. This stops the symptoms, but does not completely balance the body's hormone system. Likewise, if a patient has a group of digestive symptoms, she may be diagnosed with irritable bowel syndrome and treated with medication. This does nothing to determine why the bowel is irritated or address the causes of discomfort.

The problem is by no means limited to practitioners of traditional Western medicine. If someone with migraine headaches consults an alternative provider, an herbal formula may be recommended to relieve pain. Such treatments invite further problems down the road, since they are covering up the signals of a body system out of balance. This approach does not address the underlying cause, so the body eventually will develop another set of symptoms.

I do not treat symptoms or diseases. I simply use lab tests to determine which underlying system is not functioning properly, and then use natural therapies to restore normal body function. In the course of this process, symptoms are alleviated, and conditions such as hormone imbalances or irritable bowel disease resolve themselves. This model is not symptom-oriented or disease-based.

Most of the health problems I work with do not require a prescription or surgery to correct. They are not acute conditions — not severe enough to warrant medical intervention. I do not treat "life-threatening" conditions, but "life-ruining" ones. In other words, if you are having a gall bladder attack or seizures, you require immediate medical attention and are not a candidate for the Kalish Solution. On the other hand, people with chronic health conditions, who have been through a complete medical workup and been told they are fine, are ideal candidates for the Kalish Solution. These candidates are people who suffer from persistent, chronic health complaints ranging from perimenopausal symptoms to weight gain and fatigue. These issues can be addressed through reliable, consistently effective approaches based on sound science — without resorting to the conventional medical approach of drugs and surgery.

Changing Lifestyle

Lifestyle changes lead the list of practical and effective solutions. We all can improve our food choices, take appropriate supplements, exercise properly, improve sleep and stress patterns, and devote energy to improving our emotional and spiritual lives. Thousands of studies demonstrate the healing benefits of food, supplements, sleep, emotional expression, and stress reduction. For some people, such lifestyle changes are all that is needed to return to health, and the first stages of the Kalish Solution will guide you through them. For many people with persistent complaints, however, lifestyle changes aren't enough. For these patients, I start by doing a thorough assessment of the three body systems, using functional medicine lab testing. This is a hybrid approach that relies on laboratory analysis, much like conventional medicine, but with a focus on uncovering the underlying causes of health problems prior to the onset of a specific disease. Such nontraditional lab tests are at the heart of the work that I do. The test results allow me to design highly effective individualized programs based on natural therapies, integrating the best of scientific knowledge with natural remedies.

Most of my patients who are experiencing menopausal symptoms have significantly abnormal hormone levels, with low levels of progesterone, estrogen, or both — just how low can be determined from simple lab tests. Unfortunately, few women are offered testing for hormonal programs. Many are taking too much progesterone, often in the form of a natural cream they buy on their own. In some women, progesterone levels from these creams builds up so high that the hormone starts to convert to estrogen, creating the very problem the woman was trying to avoid. Overuse of these seemingly benign creams can induce estrogen-related problems and potentially estrogen-related cancers.

Bio-identical progesterone can be an effective treatment, provided it is used in an amount geared to an individual woman's needs, as determined by testing and as part of a program that addresses overall health. Natural (bio-identical) estrogen in prescription form also can be of great benefit, if it is likewise administered on the basis of testing and as part of a complete treatment program.

When assessing a patient's overall health, I first review her personal health history and that of her family, and then recommend the appropriate lab tests. I test for adrenal burnout, blood sugar irregularities, sex hormone levels, food allergies, and mineral levels. For women with longstanding digestive problems, I often do more extensive testing for gastrointestinal tract infections caused by pathogenic bacteria, parasites and yeast.

Diet and Nutrition

Once the lab results come back, I design a diet and supplement program to correct any problems revealed on the lab reports. I also have patients work with a nutritionist on dietary changes they will need to make. Typically, it takes three to four consultations over a six-month period to arrive at the optimal diet and supplement program, because there is no single formula for everyone. Different people require protein, fat, and carbohydrates in different proportions based on their genetic makeup, individual history of weight gain and loss, and lifestyle. Not only are proteins, fats, and carbohydrates needed in a particular combination to keep our hormones stable, nutrients within a food group can have vastly different effects. In the carbohydrate group, for example, sugar leads to a sudden rise and rapid drop in blood sugar, whereas most vegetables lead to a gentler rise and more sustained elevation of blood sugar. Remember: It is the hormonal system that continually works to keep blood sugar levels even, responding to every meal we eat.

Every patient is different. For example, a history of weight gain and loss through dieting generates hormonal problems that may require a healing diet for a period of time to restore normal metabolism. By the same token, a person who exercises frequently is going to have different nutritional needs than someone with a more sedentary lifestyle.

Creating an Adrenal Stress Profile

One of the first things I do when a woman comes to me with menopausal symptoms is to measure her stress response along with the female hormones — which means determining the impact of environmental, mental, emotional, and physiological stressors, and whether she has had sufficient rest and recovery to balance out periods of high stress. This profile includes tests for the hormones cortisol, DHEA, estrogen, progesterone, testosterone, and melatonin. It graphs hormone production over a 24-hour period, mapping out the daily rhythm of cortisol that is involved in virtually every body function, from getting a good night's sleep to burning body fat. All these hormone tests are done from saliva samples, supplemented by more extensive tests if long-standing digestive problems appear to be contributing to an imbalance. The results of these initial tests become a baseline to determine the proper starting point for a therapeutic program and against which to measure improvement during treatment.

Hidden Factors

Together, the functional medicine lab tests paint a detailed portrait of a patient's physiological functioning. There are assessments to measure the health of metabolism — whether a patient is in fat-burning or fat-storage mode. Tests are available for food allergies — an often-unrecognized health problem, addressed as part of the cornerstone strategy of determining the most healthful diet for each patient. To create a truly customized supplement regimen, I also measure for mineral levels, B vitamins, and specific antioxidants. Over many years of experience, I have discovered that the most common factors blocking a person's ability to heal using natural therapies are digestive tract problems stemming from food allergies or infections from organisms such as yeast, bacteria, or parasites. Lab tests for these issues often prove to be the key to getting a hormone program to work.

For most patients, a life-changing program calls for integrating nutritional counseling with lab testing of the three body systems, nutritional supplement programs and well-designed personalized exercise programs. These treatment options, along with emotional and spiritual change, are essential for the healing process to begin. Many studies have shown the connections between "emotional intelligence" — skill at handling and expressing emotions — and physical health. A well-known book on this is Emotional Intelligence: Why It Can Matter More than IQ, by Daniel Goleman.

Emotional & Spiritual Health

Emotional and spiritual well-being has played a primary role in the health of every one of the patients I have treated. Our feelings play a larger role in individual health than most of us realize. The importance of emotional health, loving relationships and a rich and rewarding spiritual life are often overlooked. Many people reach their health goals for a good diet, proper exercise, and sleep habits and realize they simply are missing something. These lifestyle changes are not enough to achieve and maintain optimum health.

I recently realized that the most important question I ask each new patient is, "Around the time your symptoms first developed, what was the major emotional stress going on in your life?" When this question is pursued thoroughly, I inevitably discover the death of a loved one, a divorce, the birth of a child, a job change, or some other highly charged and emotionally challenging situation. When we are under intense emotional stress, our immune and hormonal systems weaken, and we become more likely to develop a health problem, or a minor problem that is already present may suddenly be exacerbated.

In our culture, calling someone intelligent is a compliment, while calling someone emotional is usually considered disparaging. This reflects confusion as to what is most important in our lives and to our health. We are essentially emotional and spiritual beings. As the saying goes, "We are spiritual beings having a human experience."

For all of us, this is a vitally important topic. One of the key physiological effects of emotional health is reduced production of stress hormones. Stress is a natural response to many events in our lives, and the tools we use to handle it play a significant role in the development of disease.

Our emotional health revolves around our ability to communicate with others and maintain intimacy with those we love. In our culture, very few people are highly skilled and focused on developing truly intimate relationships. It requires practice and hard work. Our spiritual connection depends on our ability to see the bigger picture and realize that there is more happening around us than meets the eye. Some people discover the spiritual part of themselves through organized religion; others find it through a less formal belief system or practice.

We all benefit from exploring these areas, through attending classes or religious services, meditating, reading inspirational literature, or meeting with psychological or spiritual counselors. Achieving satisfying emotional and spiritual health will directly affect your physical health and well-being. For most of us, this is the most important and challenging step toward optimum health.

Sleep

In addition to improving your diet and exercise patterns, one of the most important things you can do for yourself is to get adequate sleep, which is crucial for physical repair and regeneration. Among my patients, I find that this is the most overlooked and neglected lifestyle change. Lack of sleep makes you tired! Lack of sleep also contributes to weight gain and poor moods. In fact, sleep, rest, and recovery are directly linked to our 24-hour adrenal hormone cycle. When the sun rises, cortisol levels peak; they taper off as the sun sets, reaching their lowest level after dark. This daily fluctuation is intended to help our bodies know when to be active and when to rest.

Ideal rest occurs between 10 P.M. and 6 A.M. Sleep during the hours of 10 P.M. and 2 A.M. repairs our bodies. Immune cells are released to seek out and destroy cancer cells, bacteria, viruses, and other harmful agents. If cortisol levels are elevated during this phase, maximum recovery will not be achieved. Between 2 and 6 A.M., sleep lets our bodies enter a stage of psychic regeneration, and the immune system is supported by chemicals released by the brain.

Rapid eye movement (REM) is a deep dream state. The alternation of REM and non-REM states throughout the night allows our minds to process emotional events from the previous day and mentally clear the slate for the next day. Without proper rest, our bodies suffer physically and emotionally. It is therefore crucial to get adequate sleep, especially during the hours between 10 P.M. and 6 A.M.

Creating a Premenopause Hormone Profile

Most of the women who come to my office are pre or perimenopausal, typically under the age of 55. Their menstrual cycles may not have ceased entirely, but they are undergoing hormonal changes and often experience many of the same symptoms as women in menopause. As I mentioned, when estrogen levels begin to drop in perimenopause, the stress hormone cortisol rises in response, putting pressure on the adrenal glands.

A woman with weakened adrenal glands who enters perimenopause is invariably faced with a difficult transition.

In treating these women, I begin by creating a premenopausal hormone profile that maps the menstrual cycle through its follicular, ovulatory, and luteal phases. The follicular phase describes the first two weeks of the menstrual cycle, when estrogen is the dominant hormone. At mid-cycle, ovulation occurs and estrogen levels peak, followed quickly by a sudden rise in progesterone, which dominates the second half of the menstrual cycle. Premenopausal hormone mapping graphs each day of the menstrual cycle, showing the rise and fall of hormones and thus providing specific indicators for hormone therapy.

Using this map, I can gauge the amounts of estrogen and progesterone a woman is producing, and compare them with established norms. I can also look at symptoms such as migraine headaches or mood swings, and correlate them with moments in the cycle when estrogen and progesterone are low, high, or dropping. Once abnormal hormone levels are detected, the solution becomes obvious, and the guesswork is eliminated from treatment.

Another benefit of this type of precise treatment program is that it facilitates resetting of the normal rhythm. I can recommend a program that exactly matches an individual woman's lab profile. After five to six months on a program, the ovaries start to produce the hormones in a normal rhythm on their own, because we have taken the time to thoroughly establish a healthy monthly cycle and normalized ovarian output. Testing of the monthly cycle also can detect double ovulation, early or late ovulation, deficiencies in the overall production of hormones, and many other subtle shifts in hormone production that are missed by other types of tests.

Since every woman is unique, her test results are like fingerprints. Even if you take a thousand women with 28-day cycles who ovulate on the same day of the month, their progesterone and estrogen levels will vary daily. So treatment needs to be tailored to each individual woman.

The month-long hormonal profile requires that the patient take eleven saliva samples throughout one full menstrual cycle. (Salivary hormone tests are not used in conventional medicine, although they correlate highly with blood levels.) A simpler test consists of taking one sample on a specific day of the month and comparing the result to the norm. The estrogen-progesterone ratio is then rebalanced using the simplest natural products, such as vitamins, minerals, and plant-based natural hormones, along with support for the digestive and detoxification systems when indicated. My patients are then monitored with follow-up testing.

Testing Menopausal Women

Menopause is usually defined as beginning one year after a woman's final period, but years of lab testing have shown that women continue to cycle internally for one and a half to seven years after their periods have ceased, having menstrual symptoms at certain times of the month even though they are no longer bleeding. Many of my menopausal patients can relate to this, since they have symptoms that remind them of when they were cycling, which appear only at certain times of the month. In such cases, responses to HRT can be poor, since it is difficult for doctors to determine how much of a given hormone a woman may need; her internal production of hormones is still varying from day to day. With accurate lab data, I can adapt an optimal treatment program for a patient as she moves through perimenopause and the first years of menopause to meet her body's changing needs.

Tailoring Treatment to the Individual

In sum, there are three important differences between the conventional medical approach to menopause and the Kalish Solution. The first major shift is toward viewing the symptoms as evidence of a systemic imbalance rather than viewing them in a vacuum, and addressing a woman's total health picture rather than just her hormonal symptoms. The second is the switch from prescribing synthetic hormones, which have been proven to be harmful, to far safer, plant-based, natural products. Finally, my approach focuses on the individual woman and her unique hormonal needs, recognizing that they change over time.

Viewing and responding to menopause in this way takes more time and effort on the part of both doctor and patient than prescribing one-size-fits-all pills to alleviate pain and discomfort. So it is not terribly surprising that doctors have been slow to move in this direction. That is likely to change, however, as more women concerned about the risks of HRT educate themselves about the alternatives and come to recognize the benefits of lifestyle changes in conjunction with natural therapies.

Exercise

As patients begin to heal, one subject that always looms large is exercise. When I start to work with patients, most are too busy and tired to exercise. Predictably, however, after a period of healthy eating, stress management, and the initial improvements that come from hormone balancing, people sleep better, have more energy, and are more productive at work. This opens up time and enthusiasm for exercise.

Exercise helps take off weight, increase energy, and prevent depression. It also can be a source of stress if not done properly. Cardiovascular exercise reduces stress, which can be helpful when done as part of an integrated health program. However, excessive cardiovascular exercise, along with a highly stressful lifestyle, can make hormone problems worse. It also can lead to more body fat by stimulating the stress response. Resistance training, on the other hand — strength training with weights — increases human growth hormone production and lean muscle mass. The increased muscle mass will, in turn, burn fat 24 hours a day. Therefore, your individual exercise requirements will depend on your hormone status and how much body fat and lean muscle you have right now.

I tell patients that designing your own exercise program is like deciding to represent yourself in court. Being an attorney requires specialized knowledge that is acquired over many years of intensive study and practice. Designing your optimum exercise program also requires extensive training in a variety of areas, and includes an assessment of your overall health to create an exercise program specific to you. Your current physical conditioning, percentages of body fat and lean muscle mass, cortisol/DHEA ratio, daily activities, and overall goals for fitness will all come into play.

Not all trainers have the knowledge to design exercise programs properly. Along with learning how to exercise, you will need basic advice on water consumption, sleep cycles, and stress-reduction exercises. Paul Chek, founder of the CHEK Institute has developed an educational program for trainers. CHEK practitioners pass rigorous exams to qualify for different levels of certification, and are trained to design corrective exercise programs and general fitness programs, as well as nutrition and lifestyle coaching. The CHEK Institute Web site (www.chekinstitute.com) lists practitioners by geographic area, so you can locate a highly trained exercise specialist near you.

A properly designed exercise program will include relaxation exercises if you are stressed, resistance training if you need to improve your strength, stretching to resolve muscle tension patterns, and cardiovascular exercise to improve overall fitness. If you have any history of injuries or musculoskeletal pain, you may require a corrective exercise program before initiating more rigorous exercise. If you are in Stage 3 of adrenal burnout, you may require some time to heal your adrenal glands before you do heavy cardiovascular exercise. Also, specific sports such as tennis, golf, running, or cycling benefit from specific stretches and strength training to improve performance and prevent injury.

When I was in my 20s, I practiced yoga five hours per day. It was the only activity I found that eliminated all my neck and back pain. I assumed that the more yoga I did and the more flexible I became, the healthier I would be. Now, 20 years later, I do some yoga every week, regular strength training and bicycling and running for cardiovascular health. I am flexible, strong, and have excellent cardiovascular health. In my twelve years of treating patients, I have worked with all types of bodies, including professional football players, hockey players, weight lifters, runners, cyclists, tennis players, skateboarders, and golfers. I have also worked with tai chi practitioners, meditators, yoga instructors, and professional ballet dancers. There is no one type of exercise that suits everyone. People are born with different body types and require different types of exercise depending on their activity levels and overall fitness goals.

Some people are inflexible and stiff. They have many muscle groups that are overly contracted and tight, and need to increase flexibility to remain healthy. This body type is at risk of pulling a muscle from excessive tension, and needs a great deal of focus on increasing flexibility and mobilization of joints. Some people have musculoskeletal systems that are too loose. They are "hypermobile" and have greater risk of injury from a trauma or an activity like running that puts a lot of impact forces on the joints. These people lack the strength to stabilize their joints. Most of us have some areas of the body that move too little and some that move too much. Clearly, someone who is stiff needs more stretching exercises, while a person who is hypermobile needs to increase muscle strength for support by using weight-training resistance exercises. A comprehensive exercise program takes all this into account. Many people also have pain and injuries that need to be addressed through a corrective exercise program. Once a person is free of pain and structurally balanced, he or she can start to achieve a high level of fitness using exercise.

Physical activity has powerful effects on both mood and energy. Research shows exercise to be as effective as medication for many common types of depression. After studying thousands of lab reports, I have come to see the importance of exercise with my patients. I have treated many elite athletes who have the same lab profiles as patients with chronic fatigue. While both patients may suffer identically on paper from multiple infections, heavy-metal poisoning, adrenal burnout, and food intolerances, the athlete's main complaint may be slower run times or waking up a little tired. In the patient who does not exercise, the same lab profile may result in chronic fatigue, obesity, depression, and a hormone problem. In my patients who are athletic, it is the amount of physical activity they do that keeps their three body systems running relatively well despite multiple insults.

Chapter Six
Gluten Sensitivity and Female Hormones

Gluten sensitivity is a common, yet little recognized, cause of female hormone imbalances that affects a significant percentage of my patients. The culprit is a molecule called gliadin, which is found in certain gluten-containing grains and causes symptoms in gluten-sensitive people. The grains that cause the greatest problems are wheat, rye, barley, spelt, and kamut. Corn, rice, millet, and buckwheat are generally considered safe; there is some disagreement about the safety of oats. In people who are genetically sensitive to gliadin, the molecule combines with an enzyme called transglutaminase, which triggers an inflammatory, autoimmune reaction in the small intestine.

Gluten sensitivity can result in a malabsorption syndrome. In sensitive people, gluten destroys the villi on the lining of the small intestine and with them the ability to adequately absorb nutrients, leading to chronic nutritional deficiencies and uncomfortable intestinal symptoms such as bloating, gas, diarrhea, and constipation, as well as other symptoms such as fatigue, depression, moodiness, and anxiety. There also may be neurological symptoms such as shooting pain, numbness or tingling of the arms and legs, and malabsorption of calcium can cause muscle cramping and tension, skin rashes, and eventually osteoporosis. Migraine headaches are another potential symptom.

People have different degrees of gluten sensitivity. If it is mild, you may only become a little puffy or bloated after eating foods containing gluten, whereas those with extreme gluten sensitivity, termed celiac disease, could wind up with significant digestive problems from eating only a small amount of such foods.

Some celiacs are diagnosed in childhood if they have obvious enough symptoms. Those who don't show symptoms at an early age are often not diagnosed. And unlike young children who show clear symptoms of malabsorption and starvation, adult celiacs frequently have vague symptoms such as tiredness, depression, and digestive problems. Standard lab tests seldom indicate a problem. Such people tend to gravitate eventually to natural health clinics that are more attuned to food sensitivities, so I see a disproportionate number of them in my practice. Many more patients turn out to have "pre-celiac" disease, a more subtle form of gluten intolerance. Such patients typically suffer from chronic health problems for years before the source is uncovered. To make matters worse, people who are pre-celiac or subtly gluten-sensitive can develop full-blown celiac disease under emotional or physical stressors such as surgery, pregnancy, childbirth, infections, or simply by overconsuming gluten.

Celiac disease can be hereditary. About 10 percent of people who have the disorder have parents, siblings, or children who share it. But because symptoms aren't always clear-cut (some gluten-sensitive people never develop the most obvious symptoms, such as digestive problems), and because celiac disease has special hormonal consequences for women, it's a good idea for women with a family history of the disease who are experiencing health problems to be screened. Other people at risk of developing gluten sensitivity include those with autoimmune disorders such as Type 1 diabetes, lupus, and chronic thyroiditis. Pre-celiac disease is quite common. Over half of my patients achieve significant health benefits from reducing or eliminating gluten from their diets.

The Female Hormone Connection

A strong relationship has been established in the medical literature between gluten sensitivity and the hormones progesterone and estrogen. Additionally, most of my patients with gluten sensitivity have an adrenal hormone imbalance, and this becomes exacerbated for patients during menopause. I have observed that serious problems often begin to reveal themselves when women with gluten sensitivity reach perimenopause. As their ovarian output of sex hormones drops, the resulting hormone imbalance is worsened by overconsumption of gluten. The adrenal glands respond to the stress of unstable blood sugar and gastrointestinal tract inflammation caused by gluten by increasing cortisol. This causes increased body fat, fatigue, and unstable moods. When gluten-sensitive women continue to consume foods containing gluten, and thus fail to absorb the nutrients they need, their cortisol levels eventually drop in the "bottoming out" of the hormone system known as adrenal exhaustion. Therefore, when women come to see me with symptoms of hormone imbalance, I always screen for gluten sensitivity or pre-celiac disease.

Testing for Gluten Sensitivity

Conventional medicine in the United States has done a poor job of diagnosing gluten sensitivity. It takes an average of eleven years for someone who is gluten-sensitive to be diagnosed, and patients typically see at least five gastroenterologists before getting a proper diagnosis. The tests used to diagnose the problem — blood tests for antibodies to gluten, and intestinal biopsy — are often inaccurate, producing false negative results. Biopsies of the small intestine are hit-or-miss, and the blood work misses some of the most extreme cases of gluten sensitivity, since people with full-blown celiac disease may not have abnormal antibody responses. Blood tests also commonly fail to discern milder cases, such as pre-celiacs.

Far more accurate, though rarely used in mainstream medicine, is saliva testing. This type of test measures what is happening with antibodies in the lining of the digestive tract rather than the bloodstream, so it can pick up on gluten sensitivity before it has progressed to full-blown celiac disease, when antibody levels might show up on conventional blood tests. Saliva testing can thus save patients years of misery. Blood testing diagnoses only one in 1,700 people with celiac disease, whereas conservative research indicates that at least one in 250 people have the problem. It is thought that many more suffer from the more subtle form of the disease.

For any test to be accurate, the patient has to be consuming gluten; the more gluten eaten before the test, the better. And while saliva testing produces more accurate results than blood tests or biopsies, interpretation can be complex. People with the most severe pre-celiac disease often produce normal results, because the immune cell counts in their intestines are low. It takes experience and often repeat testing, while going on and off gluten at appropriate times, to interpret the results accurately.

The ultimate test for gluten sensitivity is a gluten-free diet. I have my patients eliminate all gluten-containing products for 60 days, followed by eating as much gluten as possible for three or four days. Those who are gluten-intolerant will typically experience bloating and diarrhea or constipation and might feel depressed, anxious, or irritable when they re-introduce gluten into their diet at the end of the 60-day trial period. I then refer them to an experienced nutritionist who can help them follow a gluten-free diet.

The Gluten-Free Diet

The most obvious element in a gluten-free diet is the elimination of all gluten-containing grain products. For some people, this is enough to relieve symptoms, though usually not right away. It typically takes about 60 days for inflammation to begin to resolve itself. Unfortunately, any consumption of gluten will usually trigger symptoms, which can take another 60 days of being gluten-free to alleviate. Those with severe sensitivity might need to follow the diet for nine to twelve months before becoming symptom-free.

In addition to cutting out many grain products, most gluten-sensitive people must also eliminate milk products from their diet, because the cells that produce lactase — the enzyme that helps break down milk sugar — are destroyed by gluten sensitivity. This means you can become lactose-intolerant if you are gluten-intolerant. Many people figure out that they respond poorly to dairy products, since the symptoms of lactose intolerance tend to be quite clearly relieved on a dairy-free diet. Gluten intolerance is more a subtle reaction, and it takes longer to notice improvements on a gluten-free diet. If you know you react poorly to dairy products, odds are you also are reacting to gluten. Consuming milk and other dairy products can trigger many of the same symptoms as eating gluten, such as bloating and diarrhea. Some gluten-sensitive people are able to tolerate certain dairy products, such as yogurt and goat or sheep's milk cheese, whereas others cannot. Recently I have observed that many of my patients can tolerate unpasteurized or "raw" dairy products. These include raw butter, raw milk, and raw cheese.

A significant percentage of people who are gluten-sensitive are also allergic to soy products. Many menopausal women began adding soy products to their diets with news of their hormonal benefits. The gluten-sensitive often fail to make the connection when digestive problems arise.

Unlike food allergies, which can come and go, gluten sensitivity is permanent. It is a genetic autoimmune disease that will not go away over time or with treatment. The only way for gluten-sensitive people to feel better is to avoid the foods that trigger a reaction. It is never safe for them to resume eating foods containing gluten, though some gluten-sensitive people can add raw dairy products back to their diets once they've eliminated gluten.

Adhering to a gluten-free diet is a challenge at first for most people who follow the typical high-carbohydrate American diet. Naturally, our junk-food industry, recognizing a market in gluten sensitivity, has come up with a variety of unhealthful, sugar-laden, gluten-free treats. Overconsumption of these foods can cause yeast-overgrowth problems and unstable blood sugar. It's important, too, to watch out for mislabeled products. Products advertised as "gluten-free" often contain grains such as spelt that contain gliadin. All the ingredients on the label have to be examined, not just the product name. Wheat is used as a filler and thickener in many packaged foods, and can be present even in seemingly innocuous foods such as soy sauce.

The limitations of a gluten-free diet are particularly challenging for vegetarians, who are used to getting much of their nourishment from grains. A good nutritionist can help create a balanced diet centered on protein, gluten-free carbohydrates, healthy fat, vegetables, and fruit to help restore the gluten-sensitive person to optimal health.

The Craving for Gluten

One reason many gluten-sensitive people have trouble following a gluten-free diet is that they crave the very foods that they need to eliminate. When they consume the grains that cause intestinal damage, the stress causes their bodies to release natural opiates that are aptly named gluteomorphines. Hours later, the subsequent drop in the levels of these morphine-like brain chemicals can trigger a craving for gluten, a craving for that "good" feeling.

When I recommend that patients give up gluten, they often react like addicts being told to give up their drug of choice. And when they do eliminate gluten, there is often a period of temporary discomfort, thought to result from a temporary drop in the opiate levels in the brain. If you eliminate a food that triggers an opiate reaction, the resulting drop in your natural "high" can renew craving for the food in a vicious cycle of addiction. In these cases, patients may experience withdrawal symptoms such as headache, nausea, tremors, difficulty sleeping, depression, or irritability for several days or weeks after eliminating gluten. On the other hand, some people stop eating gluten and feel better right away. The level of discomfort experienced seems to be proportional to the level of gluten sensitivity present.

Within two months of following a gluten-free diet, most of the physical cravings disappear. The stronger the gluten sensitivity and the associated craving, the more dramatic the response to being gluten-free. Some people will slip back into eating foods that trigger reactions, and may need ongoing work with a nutritionist and even psychological counseling to stay on course.

Gluten Testimonial #1

Dr. Kalish: Jane, a patient of mine, had been experiencing common symptoms of gluten intolerance (digestive problems) for years, and had been to several gastroenterologists who were unable to resolve the problem. She was told she had irritable bowel syndrome. In addition to digestive problems, she complained of unexplained fatigue and muscle and joint pain, was often irritable, and felt unable to cope.

Jane: I became a lawyer when I was 35, and shortly after that I started noticing certain health issues I had never experienced before. I never was one to exercise regularly. I was always more concerned with studying, and then after that, working. However, I did lead what I thought to be a healthy lifestyle. I went to law school in New York, so I walked a lot and always remained slim because of that. After I got my first job with a law firm, I noticed my health felt very different. I felt tired all the time, I was very stressed and emotional, and my body hurt. I associated all of this with my stressful sedentary job as a lawyer. Then I started experiencing digestive problems, so I started going to gastroenterologists. I went to about four without any improvement in my health. That's when I heard about Dr. Kalish. I didn't really know what to expect from him. At that point I was convinced I had irritable bowel syndrome, and the only thing I was really hoping for was an alternative treatment.

Dr. Kalish: The first thing Jane told me during her initial phone consultation was that she had irritable bowel syndrome, and it was causing her to feel anxious and easily aggravated. As soon as she said that, I knew that we needed to look closely at her and her family's health history, because irritable bowel syndrome is often a misdiagnosis of gluten intolerance.

Jane: At first I was taken aback, because one of the first things Dr. Kalish asked me about was my family descent. While this is a perfectly fine question for a friend to ask, I wasn't sure what it had to do with my irritable bowel syndrome. Dr. Kalish explained that there is a genetic condition called gluten intolerance that can cause many of the symptoms I was experiencing.

Dr. Kalish: Jane let me know that her family came from Sweden and Ireland. Descendents of Northern Europe are more likely to be gluten-intolerant. Additionally, she told me that her father was an alcoholic, which also raised suspicion of gluten intolerance. Jane had been a vegetarian since college and had been living off grains, vegetables, and soy products. I let her know that there was a high probability that her health problems were being caused by gluten intolerance and that her tendency to eat a grain-heavy diet was just one more clue. I recommended that she go off gluten for 60 days so that we could observe her body's reaction. I explained to her that often people who are gluten-intolerant will experience symptoms of withdrawal at first, much like a drug addict going clean, and that this is normal.

Jane: When Dr. Kalish first told me to stop eating gluten-containing foods, I have to admit I panicked. As a vegetarian

I relied on large amounts of grains to survive, but I was willing to try anything. I followed Dr. Kalish's guidelines and ate no gluten-containing grains, and actually started eating chicken and fish again. Dr. Kalish told me that a healthy diet needs to be centered around protein, vegetables, healthy fat, and acceptable carbohydrates (meaning gluten-free). It was difficult at first, but after a few weeks I started to feel different. My digestive problems became less and less acute as I stayed gluten-free, and I also noticed that my stress level and emotions were feeling more balanced and I wasn't as irritable as I had been.

Dr. Kalish: Jane went off gluten and noticed extreme changes in her overall health. When we had her consume gluten after her initial two months of being gluten-free, she noticed that her old health complaints returned and she felt muscle weakness, fatigue, and irritability all over again. This was enough to determine that Jane was extremely gluten-intolerant and that it was vitally important for her to remain off gluten in order to experience a healthful lifestyle. Had we not discovered Jane's genetic intolerance, she would likely have developed hormonal imbalances during perimenopause directly related to this problem.

Jane: It's been four years since I became gluten-free, and I feel great. I have none of the initial symptoms that I went to Dr. Kalish with. I find that I have more energy and that my head is less clouded by stress and emotions. And best of all, I no longer blame my career for causing my health concerns!

Gluten Testimonial #2

Lori: I grew up in a Jewish-American family. My father owned a bakery and we actually lived in an apartment above it. Needless to say, my sister and I grew up on baked goods. We were literally living and breathing them. The smell of fresh-baked bread would waft up into our apartment early in the morning. Years later, when I met with Dr. Kalish, he let me know after taking down my history that I was probably allergic to that bread.

Dr. Kalish: I knew after speaking with Lori and learning about her family history and eating habits that she had a high risk of being gluten- and lactose-intolerant. People who crave foods containing gluten often do so because of gluteomorphins, opiate compounds released in the brain that give a "high," pleasant feeling from consuming gluten. This can lead to food addiction. Additionally, Lori is an Eastern European Jew, and people of this descent have a high prevalence of gluten intolerance.

Lori: So after I showed positive on this saliva test for gluten intolerance, Dr. Kalish suggested I go off gluten for two months. His theory was correct, and at 30 years of age I discovered that I was both gluten- and lactose-intolerant. Once I realized that I was allergic, my life basically changed, because I stopped eating that stuff. But stopping proved harder than I originally thought. Despite having good knowledge on how to control my eating from Dr. Kalish, I was still unable to do so. I knew I had a problem with addiction. It was something that I had been struggling with all my life. I remember my first binge when I was 5 — I ate an entire bottle of Flintstone vitamins. Growing up, though, I would typically overeat pastries from my dad's bakery. After I was unable to successfully go off gluten, I started going to Overeaters Anonymous (OA).

Dr. Kalish: Overeaters Anonymous is a useful resource for people with eating disorders. It is a twelve-step program modeled after Alcoholics Anonymous (AA) and has been successful for people who have a wide range of eating disorders.

Lori: The wheat would make me completely foggy and obsessed — foggy with money, foggy with relationships, with everything. I've really accepted the fact that I'm an addict. I have an addict mind, and I was addicted to food. I wasn't making unfortunate choices with food, I was a slave to it. I was obsessive in all areas of my life. That's where Dr. Kalish's program really worked. I had to understand that my addiction would spiral out and encompass other areas of my life.

Inflaming and irritating my system with gluten and sugar took a long time to repair. Dr. Kalish said it would take a year and a half to two for everything to settle, and that is in fact what's happening now. I also have a lot more energy. The fog has lifted. I am pretty much living in unmediated reality.

Chapter Seven
Food Addiction and Eating Disorders

As we have seen, food plays an important role in hormone balance. Yet the problem extends far beyond sensitivity to certain foods. Food addiction and eating disorders are nearly epidemic among American women — and are wreaking havoc with their hormones.

We live in a nation of food addicts, as soaring rates of obesity and related disorders attest. Americans are becoming increasingly overweight and underactive, and eating more foods high in sugar, fat, and calories, and low in nutritional value. A 1999 study by the Centers for Disease Control and Prevention reported that 61 percent of adults in the United States were overweight, and that

26 percent were obese. A government study in October 2002 published by the Journal of the American Medical Association gives an obesity rate of 31 percent — nearly one in three American adults. This is a problem particularly among American women, who are more prone than men to food addiction and eating disorders — which are major contributing factors to female hormone imbalance.

Food cravings and compulsive overeating are complex issues, with many causes. Food is an emotional issue for many American women, who may overeat to escape from stress, in search of comfort, or for other reasons unrelated to physical nourishment. The problem is often intensified during menopause, when the mood swings triggered by rapid hormonal change send many women to the refrigerator for solace. This only intensifies hormone imbalances, creating a vicious cycle in which women crave the very things that worsen their symptoms.

While it is important to deal with the emotional issues surrounding food addiction, understanding its physical components also can help eliminate some of the triggers of eating too many of the wrong foods.

Blood Sugar Instability

Hypoglycemia, or low blood sugar, is common among food addicts. Drops in blood sugar cause the body to release cortisol, which works to restore and maintain blood sugar levels by converting stored glycogen and fat to glucose. Low blood sugar levels can trigger dizziness, weakness, shaking muscles, rapid heartbeat, anxiety, and even panic. Hypoglycemics typically turn to sugar to assuage these feelings, but eating sweets or refined flours causes blood glucose concentration to rise too high. The pancreas overreacts, secreting excess insulin, and the blood glucose level again falls too low or too fast, triggering another sugar craving. Thus we see another mechanism for food addiction.

The sugar-laden diets fed to American children lead them to grow into sugar-addicted adults. There has been a staggering 600 percent increase in sugar consumption in the United States in the last 50 years. And even people who do not become hypoglycemic can create nutritional imbalances by consuming too much sugar.

Overconsumption of sugar has many consequences. People who load up on these empty calories tend to do so at the expense of nutritious foods, resulting in nutritional deficiencies and, in extreme cases, malnutrition — a surprisingly prevalent problem in this land of plenty. As previously discussed, nutritional imbalances can lead to, or intensify, hormone imbalances. Moreover, when the adrenal glands are assaulted by sugar, the immune system is compromised, resulting in an inability to ward off infection or disease.

Sugar also has a strong effect on mood in many people, creating a sort of high that quickly sinks to a low. Since sugar is associated with "good mood," people rush to consume more sugar, much the way a drug addict needs another fix to come back from a low once the drug's effects have worn off. This chronic dependence is much like drug addiction, with similarly serious consequences.

Food Cravings and Dependence

Foods contain chemicals that affect our moods and behaviors. Eating the wrong foods, or an unbalanced diet, promotes unhealthy food cravings and dependence. Unfortunately, sugar and refined flour (which has much the same effect as sugar and can trigger gluten reactions) are the foods people tend to become addicted to, rather than vegetables and chicken.

The foods we crave are often the foods that are the worst for us. People with food allergies — biochemical sensitivity to certain foods — tend to crave the very foods that are harming them. The common belief that we crave what our bodies need does not hold true when our body systems are imbalanced. People with imbalances no longer know what they need, and instead crave what gives them temporary satisfaction, even though these indulgences are usually followed by unpleasant physical symptoms or anxiety, depression, or lethargy. Instead of taking these symptoms as a sign that a food is bad for us, we recall mainly how good it initially made us feel, and so we seek more of it. The only way the body can recover from food allergies is by eliminating the foods that trigger symptoms in the first place.

Emotional Factors

As difficult as eliminating a favorite food from your diet can be, it is even harder to separate your eating from your emotions. Many people turn to food when under stress or feeling anxious or depressed. Just as women nurture their children with food, they tend to associate eating with self-nurturing. "Comfort foods" are usually among the worst and most addictive dietary offenders, as they are loaded with sugar, fat, calories, and largely devoid of nutrients. Cookies are invariably chosen over carrots, and the bigger the box, the longer the comfort will last (followed, of course, by feelings of guilt, self-loathing, and depression as the resulting weight gain leads to a lower sense of self-worth). The great paradox of American society is that while the media promotes the pleasures of unhealthful, high-calorie foods, it does so with improbably svelte models. Women are particularly prone to the conflict generated by these warring images because they are still judged largely on their physical appearance. They struggle with diets that deprive them of satisfaction and are doomed to failure, then punish themselves when they fail to live up to their unrealistic goals. These conditions become more acute during menopause, an emotional time when hormones fluctuate and women are more likely to seek solace in food as they witness physical signs of aging that are nowhere to be seen in the ideal models that assault us on billboards and in the media.

Weight gain is common during menopause for a number of reasons, including the widespread use of synthetic hormone replacement. Synthetic hormones promote growth (they are used to fatten cows), and one of their frequent side effects is packing on excess pounds. Many women on HRT feel unable to lose weight despite sincere effort, leading to feelings of despair and depression — and overeating as a salve.

The Diet Trap

Most American women have struggled with dieting at some point in their lives, and for many it is a lifelong battle. For most people, diets mean deprivation, and feeling deprived of foods they love leads them to crave those foods even more. Furthermore, most diets are imbalanced and built around myths. Just as there is no magic pill to restore hormonal balance, there is no magic formula for losing and keeping off unwanted pounds — and the treatments that promise such results often end up, like synthetic hormones, to have severe health consequences.

One popular diet myth is that fats are bad for you. The fact is that the body needs a certain amount of fat to function properly. Every cell wall is lined with a fat membrane that needs to be maintained. All steroid hormones, including bio-identical estrogen and progesterone, have a molecular structure based on fats, and essential fats are needed for good metabolism. Besides, as anyone who has followed a very low-fat diet can attest, it's hard to feel satisfied when fats are eliminated. Fats slow the entry of glucose into the bloodstream and lead to a feeling of contentment at the end of a meal, so you aren't left thinking about the next meal an hour later. But it's crucial to understand the difference between good and bad fats. Good fats occur naturally in organic, grass-fed meats, eggs, olive oil, coconut oil, unroasted (raw) nuts and seeds, and unpasteurized (raw) dairy products. Bad fats are artificially created, like the hydrogenated or partially hydrogenated "trans" fats found in most processed and convenience foods.

Fat

Despite popular belief, eating fat is vitally important to our health. Fats create the building blocks for cell membranes and hormones. If you are fat-deficient, you will crave sweets. However, not all fats are beneficial. Some should be avoided.

Below is a quick reference list that will help you choose your fats wisely and healthfully.

Good Fats – Choose these first

- Butter, especially raw
- Extra virgin olive oil
- Coconut oil
- Animal fats
- Nut butters
- Avocado
- Eggs
- Seeds, nuts
- Flax seed oil (unheated)

Acceptable Fats

- Peanut oil
- Sesame oil
- Safflower oil
- Corn oil
- Sunflower oil
- Soybean oil
- Cottonseed oil

Bad Fats – Avoid these

- Canola oil
- Margarine
- Hydrogenated fats
- Polyunsaturated fats
- Anything labeled "low-fat"

Another myth is that the fewer the calories per day, the better. The average person needs about 1,500 calories a day to function well. When fewer calories are consumed, the body goes into starvation mode. Metabolism slows down, so the few calories that are consumed are stored as body fat rather than being burned, which defeats the whole purpose of dieting. Many people are fooled by the initial rapid weight loss of a semi-starvation diet, which is mostly fluid loss, and become frustrated when the pounds don't keep dropping off. Real weight loss occurs slowly. On a very low-calorie diet, you lose water and muscle mass (which is counterproductive, since muscle is needed to burn calories), and your metabolism slows down. This explains why 98 percent of dieters regain all the weight they lose, plus a bonus of about ten pounds within five years. The yo-yo effect also helps to sustain a $40 billion U.S. diet industry — money spent mostly in futility and ending in hormone imbalance and a damaged metabolism.

Any diet that severely limits variety is also bound to fail. While it may seem to work initially, such a regimen is almost impossible to sustain. Boredom and dissatisfaction set in, and cravings eventually win out. Such diets also tend to lack certain nutrients and may leave the dieter feeling tired or prone to headaches, digestive problems, or serious illnesses over time.

Just as the only way to balance the hormones is by keeping the various body systems in balance, the only way to maintain a healthy weight is through a balanced diet and exercise once the three body systems are working well. However, what is balanced for one person may not work well for another. This is where biochemical individuality comes into play.

Metabolic Typing

When I see a new patient, I use food allergy testing to craft the best diet to help balance her hormones, plus a method called Metabolic Typing. This approach assumes that each person has a unique set of psychological and physiological factors that determine which "good foods" are, in fact, good for us as individuals. This assessment is based on such factors such as how we respond to food, our cravings and preferences, as well as body shape and fat distribution.

The premise of Metabolic Typing is that the effect of a particular food or diet depends on your genetic makeup. Eskimos, for example, lived virtually free of heart disease for many years on a diet high in fat and protein, whereas certain African tribes thrive on high-fiber, plant-based diets with far less protein and fat. Most people fall somewhere in-between these two extremes. The concept goes back at least 5,000 years, to the East Indian system of medicine know as Ayurveda. In ayurvedic medicine, a patient's metabolic type is addressed before focusing on his or her symptoms or disease. Modern-day Metabolic Typing combines this wisdom with scientific understanding of physiological, biochemical, and psychological indicators to define one's metabolic type.

One of the core principles of Metabolic Typing is that any nutrient or food can have completely different biochemical influences on different metabolic types. The same food that has a stimulating effect on someone of one type may act as a sedative on someone of a different type. The implication is that illnesses can be caused or exacerbated over time by eating the wrong foods or balance of foods.

In addition to genetic predisposition, environment also influences metabolism. Through excessive intake of carbohydrates, sugars, and damaged fats over the last few generations, we have significantly damaged the three body systems, and we find more and more people in the United States today with unreliable basic physiological mechanisms. Poor nutrient levels in soils, the shift toward processed, nutrient-deficient, easy-to-prepare foods, and the addition of pesticides, herbicides, hormones, and antibiotics to our food supply have only worsened the problem.

Over many years of working with patients, I have seen very few new patients with normal functioning of the three primary body systems. As we have seen, when any one of these systems is not working well, we lose the ability to utilize the biochemicals in our food properly, and cannot live up to our genetic potential until the damage is repaired. If the hormonal system is damaged, we cannot burn body fat properly, and the hormones we do produce will direct the body to store fat. If the digestive system is not functioning well, we cannot absorb the nutrients required to run our metabolism and repair cells, tissues, and organs. If the detoxification system is impaired, we cannot get rid of toxins and will have a buildup of harmful substances in the tissues, leading to a greater need for the nutrients that help us eliminate waste products.

All told, these factors lead to excessive body fat and decreased levels of the nutrients required for healthy cellular metabolism. Until these systems are restored to normal, we cannot expect a normal response to a healthful diet. Much of what patients experience in the first months of treatment revolves around repair of the three body systems. Once this foundation is established, the body can make full use of the diet right for its own unique metabolic needs.

Women and Eating Disorders

Just as women are far more prone to food addiction than men, they have a much higher incidence of eating disorders. An estimated 7 million American women suffer from two common eating disorders, anorexia nervosa and bulimia, compared with approximately a million men. It is not exactly clear when a preoccupation with food crosses over into an eating disorder, as these include a broad spectrum of behavioral disturbances from extreme dieting to uncontrolled overeating. Any degree of eating disorder can wreak havoc on the female hormones.

Anorexia Nervosa

Anorexia means "lack of appetite," but the disease anorexia nervosa is willed self-starvation. It affects about 1 percent of female adolescents and can continue well into adulthood if left untreated.

Studies have shown that more than half of teenage girls in the United States either are dieting or think they should be. They are unhappy with their bodies for failing to live up to an unrealistic ideal, and sometimes take dieting too far. Food becomes a metaphor for power, a way to try to control their internal chaos, when dieting is, in fact, taking control of their lives. Anorexics are terrified of gaining weight and obsessed with food and weight loss. They can become seriously underweight and malnourished, and in some cases starve themselves to death. They often limit their diets to what they consider "safe" foods, resulting in nutritional imbalance. When their weight drops below a certain level, the female hormones are affected and they stop menstruating. Anorexia is often accompanied by a disturbed body image and depression. Some anorexics develop the related disorder of bulimia.

Bulimia

Bulimia is characterized by binge eating followed by purging in order to control weight. While anorexia is far more common among adolescents, bulimics are often adults who may swing back and forth between periods of dieting and binge eating. Each time a woman gains and then loses a significant amount of weight, her hormonal system is damaged.

Bulimia, like anorexia, centers around the issue of control. Bulimics feel out of control while they are eating compulsively, then attempt to counteract the loss by vomiting, abusing laxatives, or overexercising. Unlike anorexia, bulimia is a hidden disease, because bulimics are often normal weight. Internally, however, they have caused severe damage to their bodies. The binge-purge cycle puts a strain on organs and perpetuates a hormonal imbalance, while overuse of laxatives causes a chemical imbalance that can be fatal.

Binge-Eating Disorder

Binge eating without purging has only recently been identified as an eating disorder. Binge eaters, like bulimics, feel out of control during their bouts of compulsive overeating, but they give in to being overweight rather than purging or abusing laxatives. Most people who suffer from weight problems have periods of compulsive overeating.

Binge eaters often overeat in secret, claiming that they can't seem to take off weight. Typically they have a history of diet failure, guilt, and shame of their overeating, and depression. Binge eating is considered the most common eating disorder, affecting about a quarter of all Americans. It can lead to obesity, and thus potentially fatal illnesses such as diabetes and heart disease. Obese women are at increased risk of developing cancer of the breast, cervix, uterus, and ovaries, and by age 60 almost one-third of them will have developed gall bladder disease.

The Alcohol Connection

My work with patients has revealed a connection between alcoholism, food addiction, and eating disorders. Many alcoholics have food-related problems. A 2002 study published in Health magazine revealed that about 72 percent of alcoholic women under the age of 25 had an eating disorder. Bulimic women in particular often have alcohol (and sometimes drug) problems. Even in the absence of a dual addiction, women with eating disorders frequently have alcoholism in their families.

While the food-alcohol connection isn't well understood, these addictions share certain similarities. Both alcohol and food are addictive chemical substances that can trap people who have addictive personalities. Both alcoholism and eating disorders lead to compulsive and secretive behavior, including denial of the problem. Women in particular find addiction to be shameful; men can be "happy drunks" or "hearty eaters," whereas overconsumption among women is seldom found appealing. So women tend to hide their problem and may fail to get the help they need.

One significant difference between food and alcohol addiction is that abstinence is not possible for food addicts. They may be able to avoid eating certain foods, but they always must control what they eat and how much. This is a lifelong struggle for many people.

Alcohol and food addiction are most successfully treated with a similar approach. Overeaters Anonymous, a twelve-step program based on the successful model of Alcoholics Anonymous, treats addiction as a disease rather than a moral failing. These are powerful, self-run support groups that offer members the assurance that they are not alone with their problem — and that others have succeeded in their quest to regain control of their lives. I have found the best choice for many people with food addiction is a combination of the natural therapies used to correct the three body systems and the spiritual and emotional support provided by twelve-step programs, therapists, and counselors.

Finding Help

The problems that exacerbate female hormone imbalances, while complex, are all treatable. Stress, depression, pain and hidden inflammation, food sensitivities, and addiction, and the many other factors that contribute to (and sometimes are caused by) these imbalances can all be improved, if not eliminated. Part II of this book offers resources for women dealing with the many issues that build throughout their lives and seem to reach a crisis point at menopause. By bringing these issues to light for my patients, menopause actually serves as a period of awakening and conversion toward a healthier, more balanced life.

Chapter 8

Chronic Digestive System Disorders

At first glance, there does not seem to be an immediate connection between the digestive and hormonal systems. But any type of inflammation in the digestive system will lead to increased production of cortisol, an anti-inflammatory hormone. Inflammation can damage the intestinal lining, impairing absorption of the biochemicals that are the raw ingredients for producing steroid hormones such as cortisol, estrogen, and progesterone, so that the body may not be able to produce as much of these hormones as it needs. Increased demand from inflammation and decreased supply from poor absorption combine to create a hormone imbalance. I have treated several thousand patients whose hormone imbalances were generated primarily by problems in the digestive tract.

People are often unaware of stress affecting their bodies. Besides the observable stress associated with life-altering events such as divorce, the death of a parent, financial problems, stress can be caused by everyday events such as a tense rush-hour commute or juggling a job and caring for children. Though largely unrecognized, this hidden stress has much the same effect on the body as observable stress, and can lead to digestive problems, which in turn have an impact on the ovaries and adrenal glands.

We saw how gluten sensitivity also generates inflammation and tissue damage in the digestive system. So do infections in the digestive tract, and with surprising frequency patients I test turn out to have chronic, low-grade infections that show up as gas, bloating, constipation, or diarrhea. Sometimes, however, even significant digestive system infections cause no obvious symptoms. What patients experience instead is weight gain, fatigue, or depression.

Unfortunately, as uncomfortable as these symptoms are, people usually learn to adapt to them by using antacids and other medications, or by avoiding foods that trigger obvious reactions. These subtle infections can rage on at a low level, continuing to damage tissues in the digestive tract. Such damage impedes absorption of nutrients, depriving the body of what it needs to function well. If you lose nutrients that help regulate fat burning, for example, you will inexplicably gain weight; if you lose those that help give you cellular energy, you will feel tired; and if you lose the nutrients that feed the brain chemicals known as neurotransmitters, or the nutrients that form sex hormones, you will feel depressed and lose sex drive. Such problems are the inevitable consequences of a long-term digestive problem.

Another consequence of untreated digestive infections affects the chemical messengers known as cytokines. These substances are produced by the body in response to infection, stimulating white blood cells to fight infectious agents. They also travel to the brain, where they induce low-level fatigue and depression, a phenomenon we commonly experience with a cold or the flu. This protective mechanism helps slow us down when we are sick so the immune system can fight the problem. Untreated, however, infections can lead to fatigue and depression that persists for years.

Of course, chronic infections also overactivate the stress hormone system, exhausting cortisol reserves. This slows fat burning, while sluggish metabolism contributes to fatigue and depression.

A final connection between the mood and the gut is in release of the chemical serotonin. This well-known, feel-good neurotransmitter is targeted by many antidepressant medications, yet few people are aware that 95 percent of the body's serotonin is produced by cells that line the intestines, while only 5 percent is produced in the brain. Damage to the gastrointestinal tract by food allergies or infections will destroy these serotonin-producing cells, and serotonin levels will drop.

In the gastrointestinal tract, serotonin promotes the motor functions of the intestines, leading them to contract and propel food through the gut in the process known as peristalsis. Lack of this muscular activity leads to constipation, and many people with digestive system problems go through alternating phases of diarrhea and constipation, usually accompanied by bloating, a cycle commonly known as irritable bowel syndrome.

Zelnorm, a new drug used to treat irritable bowel syndrome, increases serotonin levels in the GI tract, thereby stimulating peristalsis and helping to reduce the chronic constipation of people who have tissue damage in the digestive tracts. But this symptomatic relief does little to solve underlying problems.

The simple connection between chronic infections and chronic health problems has not yet been accepted by standard medicine, so these infections are rarely treated when detected. Yet, every day I see patients by the dozens with chronic health problems improve from the diagnosis and treatment of chronic GI tract infections. Patients seem to understand the connection quite readily, because we can usually trace the development of their hormone imbalance and fatigue or other chronic symptoms. Typically these symptoms coincide with a time of unusual stress. During stressful periods, immune function may dip, thereby raising susceptibility to infections, at which point a single exposure to a pathogenic (unhealthy) organism can infect a person and make her a chronic carrier.

The changes are subtle in the beginning phases of chronic digestive infection. There may be brief diarrhea, or the first occasional signs of heartburn that come and go. Once the low-level infection takes hold over the years, seemingly unrelated symptoms start to appear, such as weight gain, fatigue, and low libido. These are often accompanied by digestive symptoms, but not always. Unless their symptoms become severe, people tend to dismiss the changes as normal, everyday discomfort. Ten, 15, or 20 years can go by before the hormonal system gets involved. At this point, a woman may experience symptoms of PMS, hot flashes, night sweats, mood swings, insomnia, and the food cravings often experienced with perimenopause.

Having worked with so many patients of different ages, I find the slow, insidious progression of these low-level infections to be quite predictable. I can usually determine when the infections were acquired based on a woman's age and severity of her symptoms. On average, by the time I do a diagnostic evaluation, my patients have had an infection for 10 to 15 years. That seems to be the point when people can no longer handle the severity of their symptoms and finally seek professional help.

Parasite Testimonial

Dr. Kalish: Robyn is one of my many patients who lived for years without knowing that she was suffering from an intestinal infection. As is often the case, her symptoms did not point directly toward her problem, so she was constantly misdiagnosed by doctors seeking solutions to her symptoms rather than the cause of her illness.

Robyn: I am a 27-year old woman, and for the last ten years I have been living a very compromised life. About once a month I experience extreme fatigue, along with swollen glands in my throat and underarms. Typically this is accompanied by a low-grade fever. I consider myself to be a healthy and strong individual; however, I have never been able to fight off this recurrent condition. When I was 17, I had mononucleosis, and it was around this time that my recurrent fatigue began, so I always assumed I had never recovered from the disease.

Dr. Kalish: When Robyn told me about her condition, I immediately suspected a parasitic infection. It is not normal for mono to turn into a chronic debilitating illness, and her monthly cycle of illness was a good indicator that she was harboring a parasite, as these infectious organisms can have three- to four-week life cycles. When I spoke with her further about the time ten years earlier when she had mono, I learned that she had taken a trip to Fiji immediately after her recuperation, probably when her immune system had not fully recovered.

Robyn: Dr. Kalish mentioned that he thought it was likely that I had a parasitic infection that was contracted through drinking water in Fiji. I was skeptical, because it was my understanding that parasitic infections were identifiable by gastrointestinal problems, which I had never experienced. But then he told me that obvious symptoms are not always apparent, and that my fatigue, swollen glands, and fevers were also indicators. Additionally he told me that although digestive problems are not necessarily apparent, people typically experience a few days of discomfort directly following exposure to a parasite. When I looked back at my vacation from so many years ago, I remembered that in fact was exactly what had happened to me.

Dr. Kalish: As soon as we determined that Robyn was likely to have a parasite, I ordered laboratory tests that confirmed my suspicion, and she was finally able, after all those years, to treat her infection with antibiotics.

It's interesting to note that Robyn originally came to me seeking help with hormonal problems, specifically PMS.

As I've discussed in this chapter, hormonal imbalances often result directly from stress. As it turned out, Robyn's PMS symptoms were directly related to the long-term infection that was attacking her immune response and putting chronic stress on her body. Once we were able to eradicate the parasite and realign her hormones with a natural supplement program, both her PMS and her recurrent illness vanished.

People understandably become upset when they are told that fifteen years of digestive problems have been traced to an infection that was never identified. Most doctors in the United States are unaware that chronic digestive-system problems and hormone imbalances have any direct connection to chronic infections, because they look only at the presenting symptoms. For weight gain, fatigue, and depression, doctors recommend low-fat, high-carbohydrate diets, exercise, or antidepressants — which make most of the hormone imbalances and digestive problems worse. By this time, the patient may be told that she is simply experiencing the symptoms of aging!

From my perspective, people should get healthier as they get older. In fact, my healthiest female patients are what I call my "over-80 club." They provide living proof that you can get healthier as you age. This group, all in their 80s, are sexually active, use no medications, exercise daily, and are emotionally vital and mentally sharp. They share certain lifelong traits: They are long-term exercise fanatics, follow good diets, have had rich and satisfying personal relationships, and are intellectually engaged in stimulating mental activities. They are an inspiration to me.

Diagnosing Chronic Infections

In evaluating a new patient, I always focus on the time period when she first experienced hormonal or digestive symptoms, or when weight gain, fatigue, or depression became noticeable. This can go back as far as childhood. When I ask what the patient was going through when symptoms first appeared, she often mentions moving, traveling abroad, starting a new job, or eating a meal in a restaurant. We talk about the level of stress she was under, to see if her immune system might have been under duress.

There are usually clues as to the origin of digestive problems. Most cases involve food allergies or gluten intolerance, along with exposure to an infection-causing organism. In some cases, there is candida — overgrowth of yeast found in the digestive tract. Candida can be triggered by birth control pills, excessive sugar or carbohydrate intake, alcohol consumption, or antibiotic use.

Pathogens, organisms that cause these digestive system infections, include bacteria, parasites, and yeast overgrowth. Patients with severe health problems often have more than one, because a GI tract weakened by food allergies or gluten intolerance is more likely to contract a chronic infection. And any type of pathogen will damage tissue in the digestive system. Inflammation, malabsorption of nutrients, and the food cravings that develop from a damaged gut all trigger a protective hormonal system response that affects the female hormones. That is why it is crucial to treat the hormonal system using an integrated approach that evaluates all the body systems and can diagnose the problems in each.

I do come across patients who have eaten a good diet their entire lives and do not have any digestive problems. For these women, the normal decline in estrogen and progesterone that begins in the 30s can trigger symptoms, but far less severe than in women with a history of digestive-system problems. Such women typically respond within a few weeks to adrenal hormone programs and natural, plant-based female hormone treatments. For everyone else, a comprehensive program addressing all three body systems and tailored to each woman's individual needs is essential for restoring balance and good health.

Intestinal Environment

The gastrointestinal tract, like other major organ systems, must maintain a delicate balance to function properly. The intestinal flora, healthy microbial organisms that line the intestine, play a key role in our ability to derive nourishment from the food we eat.

The largest components of healthy intestinal flora are bacteria, which are single-celled organisms that perform many important functions. Intestinal bacteria synthesize and supplement the vitamins essential to maintaining good health. They convert dietary fiber into fatty acids needed for nourishment. They degrade dietary toxins and crowd out pathogenic, or "bad," bacteria to prevent them from harming the body. Finally, these bacteria stimulate the immune response, allowing us to fight off disease. It is astonishing to know that four-fifths of the body's immune system is housed in the intestine.

While "good" bacteria perform all these useful functions, other bacteria can cause great harm when the gastrointestinal system is not working well. "Bad" bacteria can destroy vitamins and create toxins, inactivate digestive enzymes, and convert bile or food components into chemicals that promote disease. Abnormal immune responses provoked by intestinal bacteria have been linked to inflammatory diseases of the bowel.

Interacting with bacterial colonies are colonies of yeast, which the bacteria help to keep in check. When bacteria fail to keep yeast from expanding their territory, yeast overgrowth causes significant irritation in the gut. A major cause of yeast infections is overuse of antibiotics, which kill off the bacteria needed to control yeast. Intestinal yeast infections can cause weight gain, fatigue, and foggy thinking.

Parasites are a third group of intestinal tenants, but they appear to have no redeeming value and can cause serious harm. Most people think of parasitic infection as a Third World problem, but it is surprisingly common in the West. Giardia Lamblia, a parasite that infests North American lakes and streams, causes chronic diarrhea, constipation, abdominal pain, and bloating — the same symptoms as irritable bowel syndrome. Many patients infected by this common parasite are given a diagnosis of IBS and fail to receive the proper treatment. By the time a correct diagnosis is finally made, the intestinal irritation caused by Giardia infection can be extensive and can last for months after the parasite is treated. Power Healing by Leo Galland, M.D., is a good source for further information on this topic.

Intestinal infection often goes undiagnosed or misdiagnosed for years. Failure to receive proper treatment can lead to excessive intestinal permeability, which is also referred to as "leaky gut syndrome." While the healthy intestine selectively absorbs nutrients and seals out toxins likely to cause harm, a "leaky" intestine can allow too many substances to pass through its walls. Leaky gut syndrome can overstimulate the immune response, promote allergies and autoimmunity, and allow excessive absorption of toxins. Beyond causing abdominal symptoms, it can cause symptoms throughout the body, including fatigue, joint and muscle pain, headaches, and other symptoms. Leaky gut also can be caused by overuse of alcohol or NSAIDs (nonsteroidal anti-inflammatory drugs such as ibuprofen), and gluten intolerance, as well as by infection, so it is important to determine the cause of the permeability rather than simply treat symptoms.

Part II
The Kalish Diet

The Kalish Diet is designed to improve the health of everyone, regardless of their current complaints. By following my diet, you will feel better physically, have more energy, eliminate cravings, improve sleep quality, and lose weight. In some cases, these general recommendations may not be sufficient. If you have multiple health problems, a long history of weight gain and loss, or a hormone problem that is affecting your metabolism, these changes will still help, but you may hit a plateau. In these situations, I recommend customizing the diet on the basis of laboratory testing.

In my experience, there are three "musts" in order for each of us to attain our optimum health through diet. We must

(1) determine the balance of macronutrients (proteins, carbohydrates, and fats) right for us, and choose only the highest-quality food available; (2) eliminate gluten, soy, and pasteurized dairy for two months, and (3) maintain stable blood sugar.

Macronutrient Ratios

There are three variables when considering proper macronutrient ratios: 1) genetics, 2) how damaged your metabolism is, and 3) energy requirements. It is important to keep in mind that activity level on a given day can require adjustments to your macronutrient ratio.

Genetic predisposition is an important factor, given the variation in what our ancestors ate, based on their physical environments and the types of food available. This work has been clearly explained in The Metabolic Typing Diet by William Wolcott and The Nutritional Solution by Dr. Harold Kristal and James Haig. Simply put, some people require high-carbohydrate diets to be healthy, while others require larger-than-average amounts of protein and fat.

If your metabolism is damaged, you will need to adjust your macronutrient ratios. For example, if you have chronic health problems, you will need to consume more high-quality healthy fats and proteins while you are healing. These nutrients provide the raw ingredients that aid in structural repair of damaged cells. Carbohydrates are used primarily as fuel, not for structural repair, although it is always important to have the right amount of starchy carbohydrates in your diet. If you eliminate all carbohydrates, your cortisol level will be affected, which could lead to a hormonal imbalance.

Your individual energy requirements also will dictate your macronutrient ratio. If you are like many Americans and lead a sedentary life (thanks to modern conveniences such as computers and televisions), you will want to be sure to eat fewer carbohydrates. These serve as fuel to the body, and if you are eating more than you are burning, you will push your insulin levels up, which will lead to unstable blood sugar and a host of health problems. If, on the contrary, you are an active person who exercises several hours a week, you will need to eat more carbohydrates to fuel your body.

FOODS TO AVOID

Gluten

Gluten intolerance is the most common food problem I have encountered in the thousands of patients I have worked with. It can be a serious health complaint, causing a variety of symptoms. Although not everyone is gluten-intolerant, I have found that everyone benefits from a two-month gluten-free diet, because it forces us to eat less of the processed, refined foods that contain gluten, and eat more unprocessed foods such as organic vegetables, quality proteins, fats, and healthy carbohydrates. Please see the Gluten Sensitivity Questionnaire (below) to determine if you are gluten-intolerant. People who are gluten-intolerant need to modify their gluten consumption for life. For the rest, the two-month period is sufficient, after which gluten-containing grains can be reintroduced into a healthier diet.

Eating gluten-free means avoiding all foods containing gluten, including wheat, rye, spelt, bulgar, semolina, couscous, triticale, and durum flour. Gluten can be hidden, so read labels carefully. Be wary of modified food starch, dextrin, flavorings, and extracts, hydrolyzed vegetable protein, imitation seafood, and creamed or thickened products such as soups, stews, and sauces.

Gluten Sensitivity Questionnaire

Personal Health History

Have you experienced any of the following symptoms? (Three or more "Yes" responses means you are likely to be gluten-intolerant.)

- ❑ Unexplained fatigue
- ❑ Digestive problems
- ❑ Female hormone imbalances (PMS, menopausal symptoms)
- ❑ Muscle or joint pain
- ❑ Muscle stiffness, tension
- ❑ Migraine headaches
- ❑ Food allergies/sensitivities
- ❑ Difficulty digesting dairy products
- ❑ Tendency to overconsume alcohol
- ❑ Cravings for sweets, bread, carbohydrates
- ❑ Abdominal pain or cramping
- ❑ Abdominal bloating or distention

❑ Intestinal gas

❑ "Love" specific foods

❑ Constipation or diarrhea

❑ Skin problems/rashes

❑ Difficulty losing weight

Have you suffered from any of the following conditions? (One or more "Yes" responses means you are likely to be gluten-intolerant.)

❑ Asthma

❑ Allergies

❑ Depression

❑ Anorexia

❑ Bulimia

❑ Rosacea

❑ Diabetes

❑ Osteoporosis/bone loss

❑ Iron deficiency/anemia

❑ Chronic fatigue

❑ Environmental illness

❑ Chemical sensitivity

❑ Irritable bowel syndrome

❑ Crohn's disease

❑ Ulcerative colitis

- ❑ Fibromyalgia
- ❑ Candida
- ❑ Hypoglycemia
- ❑ Lactose intolerance
- ❑ Alcoholism
- ❑ Autoimmune illnesses:
  - ❑ Lupus
  - ❑ Rheumatoid arthritis
  - ❑ Thyroid disease
  - ❑ Multiple sclerosis

Starchy foods that are allowed include amaranth, arrowroot, buckwheat, corn, millet, potato, quinoa, and rice. Oats are tolerated by most gluten-sensitive people, but are controversial as to their actual gliadin content; so be careful with oats. Avoid them for the first two weeks, then try them and watch carefully for symptoms.

Soy

Approximately half my patients who are sensitive to gluten are also allergic to soy and soy products. Part of this may stem from the ways in which soy has been genetically modified, and the frequency with which it is used as a food additive. I have my patients avoid all concentrated soy protein products for the initial two months, including tofu, tempeh, soy protein powders, and bars that contain soy protein. Most people tolerate the small amounts of soy proteins found in soy sauce or whole soy beans.

Pasteurized Dairy

Food reactions to pasteurized dairy products are easily detected. These products are pasteurized milk, cheese, yogurt, and cottage cheese — but not eggs. There are two potential problems with dairy products: lactose intolerance, which is an inability to digest the carbohydrate (sugar) portion of milk, and milk allergy, which is a reaction to the protein in milk. Pasteurization and homogenization destroy the enzymes in milk that help us digest it, the healthy bacteria in milk that help keep the gut working well, and the beneficial fats in dairy, rendering what could be a very nurturing and healing food a potentially harmful product.

While pasteurized dairy is to be avoided, raw dairy may be introduced after two weeks of a diet free of dairy. After two weeks, most people will be able to tell if they are sensitive to dairy by drinking a large glass of whole raw (unpasteurized) milk first thing in the morning on an empty stomach. If you have no digestive symptoms from doing this, then you can likely consume raw dairy products. Raw butter has butyric acid, which along with the healthy bacteria in butter helps heal the GI tract in dramatic ways. Raw butter can usually be tolerated even by people who are sensitive to other forms of dairy.

Foods Allowed

Now that I've discussed which foods you should avoid (gluten, soy, and pasteurized dairy) let's look at the foods that are okay to eat. Remember, the goal is to find the right combination of foods that will allow you to achieve optimum health by balancing your macronutrient ratios of proteins, carbohydrates, and fats.

Proteins

It is very important that you eat adequate protein at each meal. The variety of protein sources and quality are important factors. Limit protein consumption to sources that are organic, hormone-free, free-range, grass-fed, and "wild" in the case of fish. Use only fresh meats; avoid those that are processed and packaged. It is important to divide the day's total protein over the course of the day. An easy starting point to calculating the amount of protein you need is to divide your ideal body weight (in pounds) by 15 to get the ounces of protein to be consumed per day. You will need to adjust this amount up or down depending on your metabolic type, health of your metabolism, and activity level.

➢ **Beef, pork, lamb:** Eat each meat one or two days a week

➢ **Fish**: Eat a variety of grilled, steamed, baked, or poached, but do not bread or deep-fry. Limit canned tuna to rare occasions. Ask for "wild" fish. Limit fish known to have high mercury content.

➢ **Poultry:** Eat a variety of chicken, turkey, Cornish game hen, in a mix of dark and white meat. Do not bread or deep-fry. Acceptable cooking methods are grilled, steamed, baked, roasted.

➢ **Eggs:** Eat as often as three days a week. The yolk has nutrients that are denatured when cooked through, so eat eggs soft-boiled, sunny side up, or over easy when you can.

➢ **Nuts:** These may be used as a protein snack source. Raw and organic are preferable.

➢ **Cheese:** All cow's milk products need to be eliminated for the first two weeks. Choose goat and sheep cheeses and goat's milk yogurt as alternatives if your specific plan allows. After two weeks, you may introduce raw (unpasteurized) dairy into your diet.

Carbohydrates

Carbohydrates include vegetables, fruits, grains, and beans. The best carbohydrates to eat are rich in vitamins. Carbohydrates with low nutrient value should be avoided.

• Vegetables

Nutrient-rich vegetables provide an abundance of the vitamins and minerals that sustain your body. Again, quality and variety are key. Your body is most nourished with high-quality organic produce. Many therapeutic nutrients, such as antioxidants and flavinoids, are associated with the properties that give vegetables their color, so make sure you are eating a good range. Eating vegetables raw or lightly cooked helps maintain vitamin and mineral content and makes them easier to digest.

> ➢ **Green vegetables:**
> Eat an abundance of these. They are high in minerals and low in calories. Some examples include swiss chard, kale, collard greens, bok choy, beet greens, spinach, and salad greens. Dark-green steamed vegetables are superior to salad greens.

> ➢ **Yellow and orange vegetables:**
> Eat these in small portions, and always balance with green vegetables and protein. Some examples include yams, winter squash, and carrots.

> ➢ **Onions, garlic, and tomatoes:**
> Eat these as desired, unless allergic.

• Fruits

Whole fresh fruits are allowed in moderation. These include berries, citrus, melons, apples, and pears. Your best fruit choices are berries — such as strawberries, blueberries, and raspberries — along with melons and grapefruit. Avoid bananas and grapes because they can play havoc with your blood sugar; as well as dried fruit, which may contain harmful preservatives.

• Grains

Only gluten-free grains are allowed, including amaranth, arrowroot, buckwheat, corn, millet, potato, quinoa, and white or brown rice. There are now rice breads and millet breads available for toast and sandwiches, as well as rice, corn, and quinoa-based pastas.

• Beans

Beans are an excellent source of carbohydrate, and can be eaten as frequently as every meal.

• Fats

It is important to have some fat at each meal, and as with all food groups, it is important to give your body a variety. Choose from walnut, extra-virgin cold-pressed olive, sesame, cod liver, coconut, and real butter. Raw butter is ideal because it possesses remarkable healing qualities. The occasional use of safflower and sunflower oils is okay. Avoid all margarines, hydrogenated and partially hydrogenated oils, as well as canola oil and mayonnaise. Butter, coconut oil, and olive oil are the most stable with heating, but temperatures are still best kept as low as possible when cooking.

• *Beverages*

Water is the best beverage to drink. Our bodies are 70 percent water, and it is considered a nutrient, optimizing digestive function and elimination of toxins from your body. Drink two to three quarts per day of pure water. You should have at least one completely clear urination per day.

It's best to avoid caffeine, fruit juices, and alcoholic beverages, especially beer, which contains gluten. If you are a daily caffeine consumer, don't quit right away. Start by making improvements in your diet and exercise patterns, and the need for the extra boost caffeine provides will fade over time.

Food Allergies and Rotation Diets

Food allergies are becoming a more widely recognized health problem. Often it is not clear which foods are causing reactions. When I have patients who are experiencing food allergies or sensitivities, I suggest that they do a simple lab test to determine the specific foods they are allergic to, and then go on a rotation diet.

For most people, a four-day rotation interval between eating the same foods gives the best results. The food being rotated on a given day may be eaten more than once. Rotation diets are complex to follow and typically require the help of a health professional to do properly.

When Diet Changes Aren't Enough

Occasionally, diet changes are not enough to eliminate specific health complaints. When patients are unsuccessful regulating their health through diet alone, it is often necessary to test for other possible causes of discomfort. The three most common culprits are parasites, bacteria, and yeast. It is only through lab testing that these are positively diagnosed, but once they are detected, a health plan can be created that will heal these ailments and eventually result in improved health. In addition to a health plan, dietary supplements may be used, and are often a valuable way of expediting the healing process.

If you feel you might be harboring parasites, bacteria, or yeast and would like to get tested, you may set up a consult with me at www.drkalish.com or 1-800-616-7708.

APPENDIX

✦❧✦

The following is a list of supplement packages for many of the conditions discussed in this book. These supplement packages are available on my web site, **www.drkalish.com,** or via phone at **1-800-616-7708**.

The packages also include lifestyle recommendations for building health. All the supplements listed are the highest-quality products available from the nutrition company *Designs For Health*.

Insomnia Protocol

❀ Twice Daily Essential Packet: Take morning and evening. The packet consists of a multivitamin, essential fatty acids, magnesium, and calcium.

The following five are effective in treating insomnia. Start with the first one and add as necessary until you determine which help you the most.

- Reacted Cal/Mag: 3-6 before bed.
- 5-HPT 3-4 before bed.
- GABA: 1-2 before bed.
- StressArrest: 1 or more capsules before bed.
- Inositol: 1/4 to 1 tsp or more before bed.

Menopause Protocol

- Twice Daily Essential Packet: Take morning and evening. The packet consists of a multivitamin, softgel essential fatty acids, magnesium, and calcium.
- FemGuard + Balance: 2 with breakfast and 1 with dinner, 3 per day.
- Adrenotone Plus: 2 with breakfast.
- GLA 240: 2 with breakfast and 2 with dinner, 4 per day.
- Water Ease: 1 with breakfast and 1 with dinner, 2 per day (if needed for fluid retention).

PMS (Premenstrual Syndrome) Protocol

- Twice Daily Essential Packet: Take morning and evening. The packet consists of a multivitamin, essential fatty acids, magnesium, and calcium.
- FemGuard + Balance: 2 capsules with breakfast and 2 with dinner, 4 per day.
- Krill Oil: 1 capsule with breakfast and dinner, 2 per day.
- Adrenotone Plus: 2 capsules with breakfast and 1 capsule with dinner, 3 per day.
- Water Ease: 1 capsule with breakfast and 1 with dinner, 2 per day (if needed for fluid retention).

Riding Sugar and Carb Cravings Protocol

* Twice Daily Essential Packet: Take morning and evening. The packet consists of a multivitamin, essential fatty acids, magnesium, and calcium.
* CraveArrest: 1-2 before each meal, best on an empty stomach – 30 minutes before or 2 hours after eating.
* PaleoMeal: 1/2 scoop or 1 PaleoBar between meals to stabilize blood sugar.
* Metabolic Synergy: 2 capsules with each meal, 6 per day to stabilize blood sugar and normalize insulin.

Stress-Control Protocol

* Twice Daily Essential Packet: Take morning and evening. The packet consists of a multivitamin, essential fatty acids, magnesium, and calcium.
* Adrenotone Plus: 2 capsules with breakfast and 1 with dinner,
  3 per day.
* StressArrest: 2 capsules with breakfast and 1 with dinner, 3 per day.
* Metabolic Synergy: 3 capsules with breakfast and 3 capsules with dinner, 6 per day.

Weight-Loss Protocol

* Twice Daily Essential Packet: Take morning and evening. The packet consists of a multivitamin, essential fatty acids, magnesium, and calcium.
* EndoTrim: Start with 1 capsule twice daily with food. Increase after several days to 2 capsules twice daily with food, any meal.

- Carniclear: Start with 1/2 tsp twice daily. Increase after several days to 1 tsp twice daily.
- CLA: 1 softgel with each meal.

Supplement packages that treat the following are available after a phone consultation:

- Adrenal Exhaustion Treatment Protocols for Stage 1, 2, & 3
- Anti-Candida Protocol
- Female Hormone Balance Pre-Menopausal
- Female Hormone Balance Post-Menopausal
- General Parasite Cleanse
- General Wellness for Men
- General Wellness for Women
- G I Cleanse
- G I Re-colonization
- G I Repair
- Heavy Metal Detoxification
- Liver Detoxification
- Sugar Cravings
- Weight Loss

To schedule a phone consultation, please call **1-800-616-7708** or visit my web site at ***www.drkalish.com.***

Index

A

Adrenal Exhaustion *2-3, 30-31, 37, 59*
  Stage 1, 2, 3 *30, 109*
Adrenal Hormones *13, 28, 34-35*
  Mood Disorders *35*
  Weight Gain *3-4, 22, 34, 37, 40-44, 47, 73, 84, 86, 89-94*
Adrenal Stress Profile *44*
Alcoholics Anonymous *68, 82*
alcoholism *81*
Anxiety *1-5, 38, 57, 70-72*

B

Bacteria *43-45, 48, 90-92, 100, 105*
Beverage *104*
Blood Sugar Instability
  Hypoglycemia *99*
Breast cancer *vii, 13, 22*

C

Candida *90*
Carbohydrates *6-7, 29, 34, 38, 43, 62, 66, 78, 95-97, 100-102*
Celiac Disease *57-60*

Changing Lifestyle *42*
Chronic Digestive System Disorders *83*
Chronic Stress *24, 37, 89*
Cortisol *iii, 2-7, 16, 21-24, 28-37, 44, 48, 53, 59, 70, 83-85, 95*

D

Decreased sex drive *x, 1-5, 23, 30, 84*
Dehydroepiandosterone. *See* DHEA
Depression *3, 8, 12, 24, 27, 29, 35, 52-57, 63, 72, 73, 80-85, 89, 90, 115*
Detoxification pathways *9*
  Detoxification System *viii, 8, 78*
  Digestive System *6*
DHEA *2, 16, 22-24, 28, 30-32, 36, 44, 53*
  Role *31*
Diet Changes *104*
Diet Trap *73*

E

Eating Disorders *79*
  Anorexia Nervosa *79*
Emotional Health *vi, 18, 46, 47*
Endometrial Cancers *3*
Estrogen *5, 13-19, 20-23*
  Bio-identical Estrogen *25*
  Role *19*
Exercise *52*

F

Fatigue *1-4, 24, 29, 35-41, 55-59, 64, 66, 84-93, 97-98, 115*
Fats *74*
Food Allergies *43-45, 62, 72, 85, 90, 104*
Food Cravings *11, 72, 86, 90, 115*
Foods
  allowed *100*
  avoid *96*
Fruits
  Best fruit choices *103*

G

GI tract infections *86*
Gluten-free diet *96*
Gluten intolerance *8, 57, 64-67, 90, 93*
Gluten sensitivity
  Gluten Sensitivity Questionnaire *96*

H

Heart Disease *14*
Hidden Inflammation *36*
Hormone Imbalance *x, 4, 7, 8, 11, 23, 28, 36, 58-59, 70, 76, 83, 86*
Hot flashes *iii, ix, 3, 5, 21, 40, 86*

I

Infertility *23*
Insomnia *1, 3, 21-24, 86, 106*
Insulin *25*
  Insulin resistance *25*
Intestinal biopsy *59*
Irritable bowl syndrome *11, 40, 64-65, 85-86, 92*
  Zelnorm *86*

K

Kalish Diet *13, 94*
Kalish Solution *39*

L

Leaky gut syndrome *93*
Low-fat diets *6, 7*

M

Melatonin *2, 44*
Menopausal Transition *3*

Metabolic Syndrome. *See also* insulin resistance
Metabolic Typing *77, 95*

N

National Institute on Aging *14*
NSAIDs (nonsteroidal anti-inflammatory drugs) *93*
  Ibuprofen *93*

O

Obesity rate *70*
Osteoporosis *1, 3, 8, 14, 57*
Overeaters Anonymous *68, 82*

P

Parasite infection *87, 109*
  Giardia infection *92*
Perimenopause *1, 3, 31, 32, 48, 49, 51, 58, 66, 86*
Premarin *viii, 5, 12, 13, 16*
Premenopause Hormone Profile *48*
Prempro *13, 15*
Progesterone *vii, x, 2, 5, 7, 12-17, 22-27, 32, 39, 42-44, 49-50, 58, 74, 83, 91*
  Bio-identical progesterone *24*
  High progesterone level *24*
  Natural cream *42*
  Role *22*
Protein *7-9, 29, 38, 43, 62, 66, 77, 95-102*
Provera *13*

R

Rotation Diets *104*

S

Serotonin *85, 86*
Sex hormone *5, 16, 24, 43*
Sleep *x, 2, 3, 5, 23, 29, 33, 35, 37, 42-48, 52, 53, 94*

Soy products *61, 65, 99*
Stress *29, 33-36, 44, 47, 82, 108*
Stress hormone *iii, 3, 7, 23, 35, 38, 48, 85*
Sugar-laden diets *71*
Synthetic hormone replacement therapy *vii, 6, 12-17, 26-27, 51, 73*

T

Testimonial
  Adrenal *36*
  Parasite *87*
Testing for Gluten Sensitivity *59*
  Blood tests *59*
  Saliva testing *59*
Testosterone *2, 16, 44*
Three Body Systems *40*

U

Uterine Cancer *12*

W

Weight gain *3-4, 22, 34, 37, 40-44, 47, 73, 84-89, 90-94*
Women's Health Initiative *13*

X

Xenoestrogens *21*

Y

Yeast infections *4, 92*

Z

Zelnorm. *See* irritable bowl syndrome

Daniel Kalish, D.C.

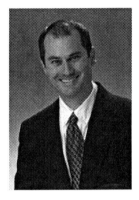

Dr. Daniel Kalish specializes in designing natural treatment programs for women of all ages with hormone imbalances. For the last twelve years he has successfully treated thousands of women using lab-based natural therapies. He also works with patients experiencing food cravings, fatigue, depression, digestive distress, eating disorders, and many other health problems, as well as people in recovery.

Dr. Kalish maintains an active phone consultation practice, working with patients worldwide. He designs nutritional programs and provides counseling to improve patients' health through diet and lifestyle modifications. In 1995 he founded The Natural Path Clinic in Del Mar, California, which offers a full range of natural therapies, and in 2000 he developed the Web site drkalish.com in an effort to reach a wider audience.

He lives in Northern California.

Notes